ELIMINATING
ADULT
ACNE
FOR GOOD

Regain Your Self-Esteem and Confidence, Avoid Unsightly, Painful, Itchy Skin, & Ugly Scarring, Without Wasting Money on Ineffective and Harmful Antibiotics, Hormones, Creams and Cleansers

By
LEIGH BRANDON

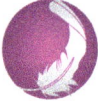

First Printed in United Kingdom 2023

Published by Conscious Dreams Publishing
www.consciousdreamspublishing.com

Edited by Elise Abram

Typeset by Amit Dey

ISBN: 978-1-915522-50-4

This book is dedicated to:

My professional teachers who taught me what I needed to learn and helped guide me to overcome my adult acne, especially Paul Chek, the founder of the CHEK Institute, and Bill Wolcott, the world's leading authority on Metabolic Typing®. They taught me so much in my training as a CHEK practitioner and certified Metabolic Typing® advisor.

I also dedicate this book to all my clients over the years who have been brave enough to venture out of their comfort zones to follow my guidance and recommendations and take on board my suggestions to overcome their adult acne.

I also dedicate this book to you! Very little fills me with as much joy as helping someone overcome their acne and in the process, improve their overall health and help improve their self-esteem, confidence and quality of life.

FOREWORD

●●●

L eigh Brandon is one of the most capable, intelligent people I've met as a teacher. Not only has he completed the extensive course study, case histories, advanced CHEK Holistic Lifestyle Coaching and CHEK Practitioner training, but he also came through CHEK instructor training with flying colours.

I've encouraged all the CHEK Institute instructors to share their clinical experience and expertise through books, eBooks, audio, videos, and so on because they have a tremendous amount of knowledge and skill among them.

Leigh has certainly been the most active among them, producing what is now a series of very high-quality books on a variety of topics from anatomy to stretching and exercise for tennis conditioning to this new book, *Eliminating Adult Acne For Good*.

In *Eliminating Adult Acne For Good*, Leigh does an excellent job of explaining what causes acne and how to use simple, natural approaches to healing this often emotionally debilitating condition.

Leigh begins the book by explaining his own painful, emotional challenges with acne and how he overcame it. Leigh has been in clinical practice for almost three decades and is a very good empirical researcher and practitioner. His offering is very important for both adults and parents, and his book can be read and understood by teens with acne problems as well.

I'm grateful to see my students producing such high-quality information, and I'm excited to announce that I give Leigh Brandon a 10/10 rating on the quality of his offering for information presented and readability.

If you want to get rid of your zits or your kid's zits forever, this book will not only show you how to do it easily and naturally, but it may also be the book that guides you to healing many other problems you didn't know were coming from the same sources as your skin eruptions!

Paul Chek, HHP,
Founder of The CHEK Institute.

TABLE OF CONTENTS

INTRODUCTION

I n this book, I will show you a step-by-step process to enable you to overcome acne, regain your self-esteem and confidence, and ensure you can live life to the fullest without any worries about your appearance and what other people might think of you.

This book will teach you a step-by-step process to follow that will enable you to take control of your health from the inside out, which will help you take control of your skin.

By enabling you to take charge of your skin, thereby regaining your self-esteem and confidence, you will never have to miss out on a social event, you'll prevent ugly scarring on your skin, your confidence around career prospects and relationships will greatly improve, and you'll have a much more vibrant and happier social life. In addition, you will no longer have itchy, painful, red, blotchy unsightly, embarrassing skin. Finally, you will no longer be a slave to your complexion.

The techniques you will learn in this book are a combination of my personal experience when overcoming acne and the teachings of many experts in the field of health and wellness who contributed to my education, either through their books or professional training and consulting.

In Part II of the book, I show you several techniques and processes to overcome your acne. Part II begins with the most important techniques likely to have the biggest effect in the long term. The techniques are listed from the most to the least likely to help you achieve great skin.

I regularly used most of the techniques I share and still do today to maintain clear skin. I went through 18 years of debilitating acne that was, quite frankly, ruining my life, but since I've educated myself, not only have I been able to take care of my own skin, but I've also successfully helped many others do the same.

There are two chapters in this book explaining the traditional medical approach to acne. In them, I clearly explain why this doesn't work for most people. When Hippocrates, the Greek physician, said over 2,000 years ago 'It is more important to know what sort of person has a disease, than to know what sort of disease a person has,' he understood the situation better than many experts today with all of the latest technology and $1,000,000 research budgets.

What Hippocrates understood was that you must treat the whole person, not just the symptoms they present with. Like any other condition, acne is just the tip of the iceberg, so to speak.

Think of it this way: you're on a lake in a rowing boat, and the boat springs a leak and starts filling with water. To prevent the boat from sinking, either you can throw the water overboard as it comes in, or you can try to block the hole to stop the water from coming in. Well if you fix the hole, you've stopped the cause. If you decide to try to pour out the water, you're just treating the symptom, and it will be a never-ending job.

When it comes to achieving great skin, it is important to uncover and deal with the cause and not just the symptoms. This is exactly what I will be showing how to do in this book. Using the same analogy, sadly, the medical approach only teaches you how to pour the water out and not how to plug the hole. The medical approach is very profitable as it usually requires ongoing repeat prescriptions.

You might only need to use the first few chapters of Part II of this book to be successful; however, you might need to use ALL of the techniques in Part II. This is because, like any health problem, the causes of acne can be due to different things in different people. We are all biochemically individual, and therefore, react differently to the same things. The same health challenges can also be caused by different factors. This is why some people do well on some medications whilst others don't. It's also why some people have different side effects on the same medications.

We are not machines! We are a complex system of systems.

In my practice, I have seen many different things that cause acne, and when the causes are eradicated, the acne clears up.

I decided to write this book as I remember the debilitating effects of acne and would like to help others achieve the same kind of success and to learn from my 18 years of mistakes and wasted time and money. It breaks my heart when I see people on social media groups asking questions about the magic-bullet product, pharmaceutical or treatment. Sadly, these magic bullets do not exist for most of us. It is important to understand that achieving clear skin involves going on a journey of education, application, and lifestyle changes that will not only help you achieve clear skin, but it will also help with so many other areas of your health and life.

This book has been written so that you can read each chapter and begin following the procedures immediately. There's no need to finish the whole book before you begin. In fact, the sooner you get started, the sooner you'll start to see clearer skin in the mirror each morning and regain your self-esteem and confidence.

However, just be aware that if your body is toxic (and just about everyone's is today), your skin might temporarily get worse before it gets better. For most, it shouldn't get worse for more than a few days to a few weeks.

As you'll see later, my skin cleared up very quickly once I knew what the cause was, but this isn't always the case. Sometimes, it can take much longer. It just depends on the causes, how long you've been exposed to the causes and how well you stick to the program.

I'm going to lead you to the water, but it's down to you to do the drinking.

By following all the recommendations in this book diligently, your skin will improve. However, just reading the book will not make a difference to your skin; you are still required to follow the recommendations.

It will require some changes to your current routine and a little time and financial investment along the way, which I know can be a challenge. However, should you choose to follow the program, you'll achieve great skin and improved confidence, self-esteem, career prospects and relationships and reduce the likelihood of unsightly scarring. In addition, others have found the program increases energy levels and helps lose body fat and increase concentration levels, as well as other benefits by following the recommendations in this book.

The choice is yours! I hope you'll join me on the path to great skin!

MY 18 YEARS OF ACNE HELL

From the age of 13, I suffered greatly from acne. Many people who have never suffered acne like you and I might think, well, that's what happens to teenagers, so it's no big deal!

However, my acne continued all through my twenties and into my thirties. As a sufferer of acne, you can appreciate how psychologically and emotionally debilitating it can be. I was teased all through school. In fact, I was nicknamed 'Zit' at school. I went to a secondary school in north London in the middle of a council estate, so I couldn't let on how badly the teasing affected me (it was a rough school), but it was demoralising. Then, as an adult going for jobs or job promotions, looking for a new partner or even when in relationships, things were a little challenging, to say the least.

You may have experienced going for a job interview, a job you know you can do better than anyone else, and it's your dream job. You wake up in the morning with nervous excitement in anticipation of showing them what you have to offer. Then—uh-oh—you feel that feeling, that intense itchiness all over your face, and you know what it is. You put your hand up to your face, and you feel the big, hot, itchy bumps. You slowly and nervously walk to the bathroom to look in the mirror to see what has arrived. When you look in the mirror, it is to find that your worst nightmare has appeared on your face, chest and back.

There were a few times in my twenties that I am sure my skin cost me a new job or promotion.

Other situations I experienced were going for a night out with bumps on my forehead the size of golf balls and my face looking like a red version of dot-to-dot! It wasn't exactly confidence-building for attracting the ladies.

Day after day, I would say, 'Why me? I'm an adult now—this is a child's problem.'

I visited my doctor several times as a teenager and in my twenties and thirties and was given antibiotics and advice on cleansers and creams. My doctor told me, 'Acne has nothing to do with diet!' which I later found out to be completely untrue. The antibiotics and creams he prescribed only made my skin worse!

I went through 18 years of not really wanting to show my face anywhere (at least on the bad days). I remember thinking that if someone approached me and said that they guaranteed they could help me get rid of *my* acne, I would be willing to re-mortgage my home; I was that desperate.

Then, in 2000, I found out about food intolerances and Metabolic Typing® from Paul Chek, the founder of the CHEK Institute, during a lecture at Loughborough University in England.

The following week, I went to see a Chinese doctor and he tested me for food intolerances. He gave me a list of foods to avoid. He also told me I had a Candida (fungus) overgrowth and advised me to follow an antifungal diet. I was also advised to stop using antibiotics (that my doctor had been prescribing for 18 years!).

After two weeks following the recommendations, my skin cleared up!

My skin is 99.999% clear these days, and I never have to think about or worry about how my skin looks. My skin is now the best it has been since before I was a teenager, and it's a real weight off my shoulders because I can live life to the fullest without restrictions. Happy days!

Later in this book, I introduce you to other people I have helped along the way to overcoming their adult acne.

HOW TO USE THIS BOOK

How you use this book is down to you. Some people like to know all the details of everything they are about to do and understand why they are doing it, whilst others just want to get on with 'the doing' and are less interested in the technical details. So, you have two options.

Option 1: If you are someone who prefers to understand why you do certain things or you like to understand the technical aspects, then it is suggested you begin with Part I of this book: Fact-Checking Acne. This will delay your getting started on the programme, and therefore, delay the time it takes to achieve clear skin, but it will probably increase your chance at long-term success by giving you confidence in the processes you will be undertaking.

Option 2: If you are someone who just wants to get on with it, you could skip Part I for now and dive straight into the Part II of the book: Your Roadmap to Clear Skin. Once you get started, you may wish to start reading Part I to help you understand why you haven't been successful prior to purchasing this book and why you will be successful following the plan outlined in Part II.

It is also vital that you follow each recommendation to the letter, as this will greatly enhance the probability of eliminating your acne for life.

Once you begin Part II of this book, it is advised that you follow each chapter in order. Please don't be tempted to skip a chapter. The order in which each chapter is written is based on my years of personal and professional experience to enable you to achieve clear skin in the shortest possible time.

So, where will you start, Part I or II?

Okay. Good!

The sooner you start, the sooner you will achieve clear skin, and there's no time like the present!

You may see results quickly—this has been the case for around 20% of my clients over the years. This is because the root cause of their acne was purely down to diet.

If you don't see results quickly, do not lose faith or motivation. Make sure you stick to the process, step-by-step. When you unlock the door to the cause of your acne, you will start to see results. It might be balancing your gut microbiome or clearing a specific toxin or two from your body, or it might be a combination of a number of things listed in this book.

Lao Tzu once said, 'Every journey starts with a single step.' Your first step to clear skin is to turn to Part I or Part II and get started!

In Part III of this book, I have included Putting It All Together, a step-by-step plan outlining the order in which to complete each task, how long you need to spend on each task and when it's the ideal time to begin the next task. This section does not include how to complete the tasks, as that information is included in Part II.

This book might possibly be the most comprehensive approach to eliminating acne you will find outside of hiring a very well-qualified and skilled professional who, like me, has walked that journey and is now helping others to do the same.

Now, it's time to turn to Part I or Part II and get started.

PART I

FACT-CHECKING ACNE

THE GOOD, THE BAD AND THE UGLY

'There is no evidence that diet plays a role in acne.'[1]

I n this chapter, I outline what is good, bad and ugly about the current medical approach to acne.

The Current Medical Acne Paradigm

If you ask most medical doctors, they will tell you that acne is formed by a combination of the following factors:

- excess androgens (male hormones)
- excess sebum secreted from sebaceous glands due to excess androgens
- excess sebum secreted to moisturise dry skin
- blockage of the pores around hair follicles due to excess sebum
- build-up of dead skin in hair follicles causes blockages and a further increase in sebum production to clear the blockages

---

[1] 'Overview Acne,' 2017

- the bacteria *Cutibacterium acnes* (formerly known as *Propioni-bacterium acnes*), which lives in the pores, begin to feed and flourish on the blocked sebum and dead skin
- inflammation due to bacterial infection

DEFINITION:

According to the *Merriam-Webster Dictionary,* **Sebum** is the fatty lubricant matter secreted by sebaceous glands of the skin.

Sebaceous glands *are* any of the small sacculated glands lodged in the substance of the derma, usually opening into the hair follicles and secreting an oily or greasy material composed in great part of fat, which softens and lubricates the hair and skin.

The problems are not so much the increase in androgens, blocked pores or the bacteria building up on the dead skin but what is causing the increase in androgens, blocked pores, infections and inflammation.

Not addressing the underlying cause is why skin creams and cleansers do not work for most people in the long run. They merely mask the symptoms if you're lucky. You might be able to keep clearing the skin, but the underlying cause is still there.

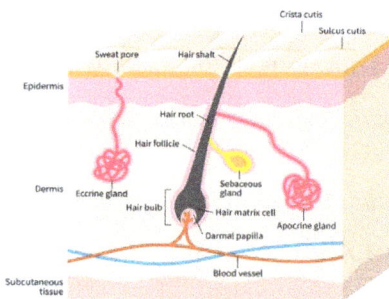

Doctors sometimes give women the contraceptive pill to balance hormones, but what is causing the hormones to be out of balance in the first place?

Unless these answers are found and dealt with, the problem (acne) will bubble up under the surface and rear its head whenever it likes. Acne is not

Diagram depicting the skin layers, including the Sebaceous gland.

caused by a deficiency in cleansing creams, antibiotics or a lack of synthetic hormones.

According to Dr William Kellas and Dr Andrea Dworkin, in their book, *Thriving in a Toxic World*, acne can be caused by too much cadmium, mercury, sugar, microorganisms or allergies, and I will tackle each of these subjects throughout the book.

Research[2, 3, 4, 5, 6, 7, 8, 9, 10] suggests there is a link between an increase in the hormone insulin and insulin-like growth factor-1 (IGF-1) and acne. Research suggests these increased hormone levels can cause acne by:

- increasing sebum production,
- increasing the generation of skin cells and
- dead skin cells sticking together.

The hypothesis suggests that a faster generation of skin cells causes more dead skin cells to be pushed through the skin's pores. When dead skin cells stick together, they are pushed through the skin's pores in large quantities rather than one skin cell at a time. Then, you have a lot of sticky sebum, which is likely to lead to blocked pores and breakouts.

One thing I must also make clear is that your skin is your largest organ, and it is an organ of detoxification. Dr Ben Johnson of Osmosis Beauty is unconvinced acne is caused by bacterial infections (as

---

[2] Melnik, 2011

[3] Danby, 2010

[4] Jung et al, 2010

[5] Smith et al, 2008

[6] Smith et al, 2007a

[7] Smith et al, 2007b

[8] Cordain et al, 2003

[9] Borgia et al, 2004

[10] Slayden et al, 2001

described by the medical establishment) and believes acne is caused by the skin purging toxins from the body.[11]

Your skin is a good barometer of how well you are doing on the inside. In my view, acne is a condition caused by an imbalance of one or more of the body's systems. I will teach you how to balance your body's systems, thereby improving your skin. This is exactly how my clients and I did it and how we maintain it.

I opened this chapter with a quotation from the UK's National Health Service, stating, 'There is no evidence that diet plays a role in acne'—is it true there is no evidence that diet plays a role in acne? Find out in Chapter 2!

The Effects of Traditional Medical Acne Treatments

In this section, I show you the common medical approaches to acne, their positive and negative effects and why they are still recommended. In other words, The Good, The Bad and The Ugly!

There are four main medical approaches that tend to be used for acne:

1. Antibiotics
2. Combined contraceptives for females
3. Other hormone treatments
4. Topical creams and cleansers

Antibiotics

Antibiotics used for acne include:

- erythromycin
- tetracycline
- doxycycline
- minocycline

---

[11] Osmosis Beauty, 2020

Whilst antibiotics can be effective in the short term, long-term use can be detrimental to your overall health. If the antibiotics are effective, you must stop taking them long term because it is not safe to continue long-term so; in almost all cases, the acne will just bounce back once they are stopped.

If antibiotics are used long-term (as I did), as well as not always being effective, they often make the acne worse, and they can cause antibiotic resistance and damage to the gut microbiome. Antibiotic resistance can cost you your life if antibiotics don't work when you need them to keep you alive after you are in a serious accident or need surgery, for instance.

As well as killing the Cutibacterium acnes, antibiotics also kill the commensal (beneficial) bacteria that arguably play the most important role in our overall health. Almost all disease is linked with dysbiosis (imbalanced bacteria).

Antibiotics leave the door wide open to pathogenic bacteria and fungi, which may also cause acne and many other diseases. Studies have shown those who use topical and oral antibiotics are three times as likely to show an increase of bacteria in the throat and tonsils compared with non-users.[12]

Long-term use of antibiotics in acne treatment is also associated with an increase in upper respiratory infections and skin bacteria and has been shown to affect blood sugar levels, as well.[13]

We need to be aware of the potential consequences when we use antibiotics and carefully weigh the risks and benefits.

Combined Contraceptives

Contraceptive pills are given to women to reduce the level or effect of androgens in the body. Though they tend to be effective in reducing

[12] 'Doctors turning,' 2019
[13] 'Doctors turning,' 2019

acne whilst in use, the acne tends to worsen when the contraceptive is stopped.

Taken over the long term, contraceptives have been linked with[14]

- blood clots:
    - o   deep vein thrombosis
    - o   pulmonary embolus
    - o   stroke
- heart attack
- high blood pressure
- breast, cervical, endometrial, ovarian, bowel and liver cancers
- osteoporosis
- gallbladder disease
- zinc deficiency

Other Hormone Treatments

Isotretinoin/Accutane:

Isotretinoin (formerly known as Accutane) is only given for severe acne when all other medical avenues have been tried. Sadly, it is used quite regularly as the other treatments are often ineffective long term.

Isotretinoin works by unclogging pores, reducing the stickiness of keratinocytes inside the follicle, slowing down sebum production and shrinking sebaceous glands.

This can be effective, but at what cost?

Side Effects:[15]

- Your skin may become very dry and sensitive to sunlight during treatment. Using lip balm and moisturisers will help.

---

[14] 'Combined Pill,' 2020

[15] 'Isotretinoin capsules,' 2022

- It's very important not to become pregnant while using isotretinoin capsules and for at least one month after stopping. This is because isotretinoin can harm an unborn baby.

- If you become depressed or think about harming yourself while taking isotretinoin, stop taking the medicine and tell your doctor straight away.

- Your skin may become more sensitive to sunlight.

- You may experience dry eyes.

- You may experience a dry throat.

- You may experience a dry nose and nosebleeds.

- You may suffer from headaches and general aches and pains.

- You may experience anxiety, aggression, violence, changes in mood or suicidal thoughts. These can be signs of depression or other mental health problems.

- You may feel severe pain in your stomach with or without diarrhoea and feeling or being sick (nausea or vomiting). These can be signs of a serious problem called pancreatitis.

- You may have bloody diarrhoea. This may be a sign of gastrointestinal bleeding.

- You may have a serious skin rash that peels or has blisters. The skin rash may come with eye infections, ulcers, fever or headaches.

- You may find it difficult to move your arms or legs, have painful, swollen or bruised areas of the body or dark pee. These can be signs of muscle weakness.

- Your skin or the whites of your eyes might turn yellow; you might have difficulty peeing or feel very tired. These are signs of liver or kidney problems.

- You may have a bad headache that doesn't go away and makes you feel sick or be sick.

- There may be sudden changes in eyesight, including not seeing as well at night.

Isotretinoin capsules can sometimes cause depression or make it worse and *can* even make *some* people feel suicidal.

Spironolactone:

Spironolactone is typically prescribed for high blood pressure, heart failure and swelling, but it is also used to reduce acne symptoms in women. It works by slowing the production of androgens (aldosterone).

Common side effects of spironolactone for girls and women can include:[16]

- breast tenderness and/or breast enlargement
- painful and/or irregular periods, as well as vaginal bleeding after menopause
- hair loss
- photosensitivity (sensitivity to UV rays from the sun and other light sources)
- nausea and vomiting
- drowsiness

Co-cyprindiol:

Co-cyprindiol is another hormone treatment prescribed to women for severe acne that doesn't respond to antibiotics. It helps to reduce the production of sebum.

Side effects of co-cyprindiol include:[17]

- bleeding and spotting between periods
- headaches

---

[16] 'Side effects of spironolactone,' 2022

[17] 'Treatment: Acne,' 2017

- sore breasts
- mood changes
- low libido
- weight gain or weight loss
- blood clots
- breast cancer

Again, co-cyprindiol does not address the 'why' of hormone imbalances; it only attempts to mask the symptoms.

Topical treatments:

Benzoyl Peroxide:

Benzoyl peroxide works as an antiseptic to reduce the amount of bacteria on the surface of the skin.

It also helps reduce the number of whiteheads and blackheads and has an anti-inflammatory effect. Benzoyl peroxide is advertised as a six-week treatment. Common side effects of benzoyl peroxide are:[18]

- dry and tense skin
- a burning, itching or stinging sensation
- some redness and peeling of the skin
- permanent staining when it comes into contact with carpets

Salicylic Acid:

Salicylic acid works to dissolve the dead skin cells clogging the pores. It can cause:[19]

- skin irritation
- skin dryness
- skin tingling or stinging

---

[18] 'Treatment: Acne,' 2017

[19] 'Treatment: Acne,' 2017

- itching
- peeling skin
- hives

Azelaic Acid:

Azelaic acid is often used as an alternative treatment instead of benzoyl peroxide or topical retinoids. It works by getting rid of dead skin and killing bacteria.

The side effects of azelaic acid include:[20]

- burning or stinging skin
- itchiness
- dry skin
- redness of the skin

My Confession

I need to be completely transparent here: my clients have reported side effects caused by my program. My clients report:

- reduced body fat
- more energy
- calmer tummy
- better bowel movements
- sleeping better
- improved concentration
- more confidence
- better social life
- less anxiety
- less stress
- feeling better about themselves

[20] 'Treatment: Acne,' 2017

- not needing to wear tons of make-up
- they are happier!!!

Don't worry—I will show you how to achieve these results in Part II of this book.

When you look at the side effects from medical solutions currently being offered by chemical/pharmaceutical/medical establishments and compare them to the side effects my clients report using a natural, holistic approach, I hope you will begin to understand the risk-benefit ratio existing between the two approaches.

One approach, which is often ineffective, has been known to cause antibiotic resistance, blood clots, heart attacks, high blood pressure, cancer, strokes, headaches, general aches and pains, anxiety, aggression, violence, changes in mood, suicidal thoughts, mental health problems, severe stomach pain, nausea or vomiting, pancreatitis, gastrointestinal bleeding, serious skin rashes, breast tenderness and/or breast enlargement, painful and/or irregular periods, vaginal bleeding, hair loss, low libido, weight gain, blood clots, dry and tight skin, burning, itching or stinging skin, redness and peeling of the skin and much more.

The other approach (that I use), in addition to improving acne, has been shown, in some cases, to also cause reduced body fat, more energy, a calmer tummy, better bowel movements, better sleep, better concentration, more confidence, an improved social life, the reduced need to wear make-up, feeling less anxious, less stressed, and better about themselves and feeling happier overall!!!

So, in terms of looking at the risk-benefit ratio, which approach would you prefer?

I'm not here to tell you what you should do but rather to help educate you so you can make the right decisions for you. I'm guessing that if you are reading this book, you are already aware of the ineffectiveness of the medical approach, have possibly experienced negative side effects and are ready to try something different that has already worked for many other people.

Why Is the Medical Approach Allowed?

I am often confronted by people asking me why the medical approach *is* allowed to continue and why don't doctors know more or do more.

Sadly, it comes down to market forces and economics. Whilst we are led to believe the medical establishment and their colleagues in the pharmaceutical industry have a common goal to help people achieve optimal health, sadly, this is not the case.

I am not, for one second, suggesting the people working in these industries are bad or are consciously doing harm—I am aware that in some circumstances, they do amazing things. However, money talks!

What you may or may not be aware of is that with their huge financial clout, the pharmaceutical industry has a lot of influence in several sectors. Firstly, they heavily subsidise the education of medical doctors and in return, have almost complete control over the curriculum.

Pharmaceutical companies also have a major influence over the organisations that are supposed to regulate them. The table below[21] displays how much funding for pharmaceutical regulators comes from the very companies they are supposed to regulate in each county. As you see, in the case of Australia, this is as much as 96%. It would be naïve to think these companies invest that much money without expecting a return on their investment. Some might even suggest this is a case of the fox guarding the chicken coop.

Sadly, corruption is rife when it comes to pharmaceutical regulation. There is a constant revolving door of regulators authorising products—who join the companies standing to make billions from the products they approve and often without proper safety testing—with the reward of a multi-million-dollar salary.

Through the lobbying of government officials and politicians, pharmaceutical companies have a huge influence over government policies to maximise their profits. According to *Statista*, in 2022, the

---

[21] Demasi, 2022

Table 1 How the regulators compare

	Australia TGA	Europe EMA	UK MHRA	Japan PMDA	USA FDA	Canada HC
Budgets and fees						
Proportion of budget derived from industry°	96%	89%	86%	85%	65%	50.5%
Total annual budget†	AU$170m (£95m)	€386m (£331m)	£159m	¥29.1bn (£175m)	US$6.1bn (£5bn)	C$2.7bn (£1.7bn)
Transparency, COIs, and data						
Proportion of covid-19 vaccine committee members that declared financial COIs	50%	3%	32%	75%	<10%	0%
Declared COIs available as public information	No	Yes	Yes	Yes	Yes	No
Regulator routinely receives patient level datasets*	No	No	No	Yes	Yes	No
Drug approvals						
Proportion of decisions to approve	94%	88%	98.5%	Not disclosed	69%^ ...#	83%

pharmaceutical industry gave $306,000,000 to US politicians alone.[22] Not a bad gig if you're a US politician without ethics or morals!

In addition, pharmaceutical companies and their government agency partners control research grant funding. This means that research is only performed in order to make their products look good and further their business interests and profit margins. This was illustrated very well in Robert F Kennedy Jr's book, *The Real Anthony Fauci: Bill Gates, Big Pharma, and the Global War on Democracy and Public Health*.[23]

Having performed a lot of research on acne, I've discovered that much research is performed on medical products. Whilst there are some research papers on nutrition and acne, there is little profit to be made from nutritional advice, and due to the huge expense of research— meaning there is no profit to be made—the research in this area is relatively limited.

I also noticed that, as is the case with most research, studies performed on acne are rarely—if ever—longer than 6-12 weeks. My own

---

[22] 'Leading lobbying,' 2023
[23] 2021

experience suffering from acne and using pharmaceutical products is that I achieved a short-term reduction in symptoms, but in the long term, they made my acne worse. A research paper might suggest that a particular product is effective; however, if the study was followed up at one-, five- or 10-year intervals, chances are there would be a completely different outcome.

Very sadly, our medical/pharmaceutical industry, first and foremost, has a responsibility to its shareholders. The shareholders of any business are there to make money. That is what a commercial enterprise does, or it would be a charity. So what we have is a medical system whose priority is to make as much profit as possible and continue to increase the growth of their profits year on year.

What we do not have is a medical system that prioritises the health outcomes of its patients. The pharmaceutical industry sees you as a 'consumer'. As an industry that exists to make as much money as possible, prolonged illnesses and diseases are how they make their money. This means that if they can keep you in a state of dis-ease, they can continue to make money from you. The longer you have acne and the more you try their products, the more money they make. If you completely cure your acne, you are no longer profitable for them.

What you might also find interesting is that pharmaceutical companies have received the largest criminal fines in history, adding up to several billions of dollars for making misleading claims about their products' efficacy and safety, for fraud, and for bribing medical doctors, to name but a few infractions. These companies are so rich and powerful that they can put these huge fines down to marketing costs and still make huge profits.[24, 25, 26]

I previously mentioned that pharmaceutical companies have great influence over the curriculum of medical degrees. A large proportion of medical training includes the study of symptomology and

[24] 'Pfizer to pay', 2009

[25] Khan & Thomas, 2010

[26] Costinescu, 2009

pharmacology. Doctors are trained that if they see a certain symptom, there are options as to which pharmaceutical interventions they might use to treat that symptom. The problem with this approach is it encourages dependence on medication and does not attempt to deal with the causes of the dis-ease in the first place.

If you present with acne, you might be offered antibiotics and benzoyl peroxide cream for your acne, but that does not deal with the cause. Even if the treatment works in the long term, which is unlikely, you are likely to suffer negative side effects and be reliant on these products for the rest of your life, along with other pharmaceutical products prescribed to deal with the side effects of the acne medications. What this does is create a great repeat business for the companies making the products without helping you overcome your acne in the long term.

I have sympathy for medical doctors. I believe most of them are genuinely trying to help, and there are a small minority of fantastic doctors who go beyond their training to provide highly effective service. Sadly, for most doctors, their training has let them down. When speaking to several doctors in recent years, they tell me that in seven years of medical school, they received between zero and four hours of nutrition training. This might be why the UK's National Health Service still believes there is no link between diet and acne and why they don't really know how to treat patients with acne with any great success.

Chapter summary/Key takeaways

In summary:

- The medical establishment teaches us there is no evidence that diet is related to acne.

- There are multiple biological and chemical steps involved in the formation of acne.

- Androgens (male hormones), insulin and Insulin-like Growth Factor-1 (IGF-1) are thought to be involved in the cause of acne.

- Excess sebum production, blocked skin pores, proliferation of the C. acnes bacteria, and inflammation may lead to acne formation.

- Skin creams, lotions and antibiotics tend not to work for most people as they do not get to the cause of acne.

- The skin is the largest detoxification organ, so acne can be a barometer of imbalance on the inside of your body.

- Whilst there are some successful outcomes with current medical approaches to acne, they do not work more often than not, and there are often serious side effects, including death, that can happen when using these products.

- Following a natural, holistic approach that has proven successful treats the underlying causes of acne and often comes with several positive side effects.

- The medical establishment and its regulators are heavily controlled by corporations whose main objective is to make money. The training of medical doctors is heavily controlled by these corporations, and the outcomes of patients are not a high priority for corporations. Their priority, first and foremost, is to their shareholders.

- There is much money to be made in keeping people in a state of dis-ease, and the healing of states of dis-ease would be harmful to these powerful corporations. Sadly, the sufferers of acne get caught in the crossfire.

In the next chapter, you will learn what most doctors don't know: what really causes acne.

WHAT REALLY CAUSES ACNE?

'So far research has not found any foods that cause acne.'[27]

To really understand what causes acne, we need to take a dive into some technical information. I will attempt to make it as easy to understand as possible (although this section will get a little technical).

In this chapter, I outline important topics such as:

- the skin's acid-alkaline balance or pH levels,

- the skin's microbiome and the link between the gut and the skin, commonly referred to as 'The Gut-Skin Axis',

- fungal acne,

- the four major causes of acne (by consensus),

- the mTOR Pathway and

- foods shown by research to cause acne.

---

[27] 'Overview: Acne,' 2017

The Skin's pH

Before I delve straight into talk about the skin's pH, I thought it best to define pH[28], just so we are on the same page.

> In chemistry, **pH**, historically denoting the 'potential of hydrogen' is a scale used to specify the acidity or basicity of an aqueous solution.
>
> Acidic solutions (solutions with higher concentrations of H^+ ions) are measured to have lower pH values than basic or alkaline solutions.

Now that we have cleared that up, let us begin.

Our skin helps us protect the inside of our bodies from the external environment and preserve the loss of water from our internal environments.[29] Our skin creates a protective barrier against bacteria, viruses, and other contaminants and produces an acid mantle on the outermost layer of the skin, the stratum corneum.[30, 31] The stratum corneum is comprised of several substances—such as corneocytes, lipids (such as ceramides), fatty acids and cholesterol—all of which form a multilayer barrier.[32, 33]

While the pH of healthy skin ranges from around four to six (slightly acidic), inflamed and diseased skin tends to exhibit an

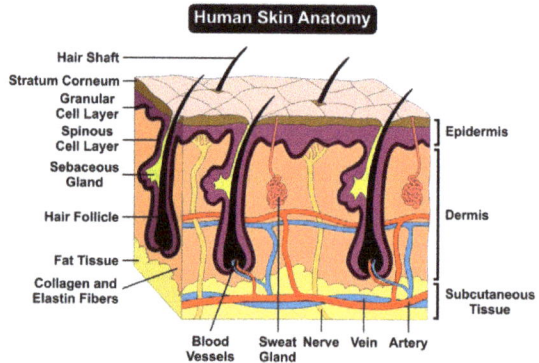

Human Skin Anatomy

Hair Shaft
Stratum Corneum
Granular Cell Layer
Spinous Cell Layer
Sebaceous Gland
Hair Follicle
Fat Tissue
Collagen and Elastin Fibers
Epidermis
Dermis
Subcutaneous Tissue
Blood Vessels   Sweat Gland   Nerve   Vein   Artery

---

[28] 'pH,' 2001

[29] Blaak et al., 2017

[30] Borgia et al., 2004

[31] Bouwstra, 2006

[32] Bouwstra, 2006

[33] Kim et al., 2009

increased pH (alkaline).[34, 35, 36] Changes in skin pH play a role in the pathogenesis of wrinkles and skin diseases, so it's important to pay attention to our skin's pH if we wish to overcome acne.[37]

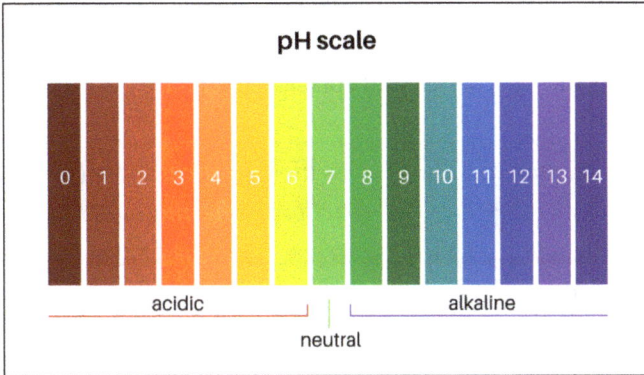

The human body has pH levels ranging from one to eight, (one being the most acidic, seven being neutral, and 14 being the most alkaline). pH levels differ in different parts of the body. The following are some examples of average pH levels in the body:[38]

- stomach acid: pH 1-1.5
- stratum corneum (top layer of skin): pH 4-6
- blood: pH 7.35-7.45
- urine: pH 6.5-8

The skin's pH is maintained by metabolic and cellular processes that regulate protons, including a sodium/hydrogen exchanger, free fatty acids made

[34] Kim et al., 2018

[35] Proksch, 2018

[36] Eo et al., 2016

[37] Youn, 2013

[38] Ali & Yosipovitch, 2013

from phospholipids, free amino acids created by filaggrin degradation, and epidermal lactate produced by lactate dehydrogenase.[39, 40, 41]

This means that the skin's pH is maintained by several processes involving protons in the cells, minerals, fats and amino acids from skin cells and enzymes on the skin's surface.

A range of enzymes are crucial in maintaining a low pH, including lipases, glycoside hydrolases and sphingomyelinases.[42]

> **Enzymes**[43] *are proteins that act as biological catalysts (biocatalysts). Catalysts accelerate chemical reactions. The molecules upon which enzymes may act are called substrates, and the enzyme converts the substrates into different molecules known as products.*

However, when skin pH increases, these enzymes are not fully activated; instead, enzymes involved in the degradation of the stratum corneum are enhanced, leading to a breakdown in skin barrier integrity.[44]

The acidic pH of skin plays several important roles, including:[45]

- creating a physical barrier
- preventing over-colonisation of bacteria and yeasts, including Cutibacterium acnes
- lipid synthesis and aggregation (making and adding lipids (fats))
- epidermal desquamation (skin shedding)
- ceramide metabolism (**ceramides** are a family of waxy lipid molecules).

---

[39] Kim et al., 2018

[40] Ali & Yosipovitch, 2013

[41] Jang et al., 2016

[42] Kim et al., 2018

[43] 'Enzyme,' 2001

[44] Kim et al., 2018

[45] Ali & Yosipovitch, 2013

Both endogenous (internal) and exogenous (external) factors influence the skin's pH.

Some endogenous factors cannot be changed, but exogenous factors give you many options when trying to shift the pH of your skin.

Endogenous factors include age, region of the body, ethnicity and gender, whilst exogenous factors include climate, products used on the skin, microbiome and diet.

In the modern world, we use soaps and shampoos to clean our bodies of bacteria and unwanted smells. However, soaps and shampoos are generally alkaline, and their use causes an increase in our skin's pH.[46] Washing with water can cause a rise in pH that will take six hours to normalise, and the use of alkaline soaps raises pH even higher.

In one study, a topical lotion with 1% sodium lauryl sulphate (SLS) was added to the skin (SLS is an irritant to the skin) to see the impact pH would have on the ability to tolerate irritation. SLS impaired the skin barrier overall but had the greatest impact on pH8 skin. Researchers suggest that acidic skin is better able to tolerate external irritants and stress than alkaline skin.[47]

A person's age has an impact on pH, with the first month of life, as well as the elderly, having a higher average pH than other ages. Ageing skin is known to have a higher pH as well as a lower stratum corneum lipid content, and excessively dry skin is a common problem amongst the elderly.[48, 49] It is believed that a higher pH activates enzymes involved in barrier lipid degradation, such as ceramidase.[50]

Some studies have shown that men tend to have a slightly lower pH than women overall.[51, 52, 53]

---

[46] Takagi et al., 2015

[47] Kim et al., 2009

[48] Blaak et al., 2017

[49] Jang et al., 2016

[50] Eo et al., 2016

[51] Prakash et al., 2017

[52] Youn et al., 2013

[53] Luebbberding et al., 2013

Another study of 300 healthy males and females from age 20 to 74 showed that, on average, men's pH was below five and women's pH was higher than five.[54]

Sebum production in males is significantly higher than in women, and Trans Epidermal Water Loss (TEWL) was lower in men than women of the same age, meaning their skin maintains more of the crucial moisture.[55] Sebum levels in men are 20% greater on the forehead and 70% greater on the cheeks on average than that of women.[56]

Sebaceous gland activity in males has been shown to be relatively constant regardless of age, whereas in females, a reduction in sebum production occurs around the age of 40.[57]

The acidity of the skin varies depending on the location on the body, as well as 'physiologic holes of the acid mantle' that exist in certain locations.[58] Areas like the armpit, groin and below the breasts tend to have a higher pH compared to other locations. Odour-causing bacteria can thrive in these zones, so many deodorants contain citrates, which reduce pH to make it inhospitable to these bacteria.[59]

Candida also thrives in this more alkaline environment, often appearing in intertriginous zones, which are the areas the skin might touch or rub, like the insides of elbows, the backs of knees and under the breasts.[60]

Different areas on the same part of the body can have different pH levels. In one study of the T-zone (forehead, nose and chin) and U-zone (both cheeks), it was found that the average pH of the T-zone was higher than the U-zone at 5.66 versus 5.53 respectively.[61]

---

[54] Luebberding et al., 2013

[55] Luebberding et al., 2013

[56] Luebberding et al., 2013

[57] Luebberding et al., 2013

[58] Prakash et al., 2017

[59] Eo et al., 2016

[60] Eo et al., 2016

[61] Youn et al., 2013

Acne is a skin disease known to involve a disrupted skin barrier and increased pH.[62] Researchers studied 200 patients with acne and 200 controls with healthy skin. Normal pH was defined as 4.5 to 5.5 for women and four to 5.5 for men.[63]

They found that participants in the control group had an overwhelmingly normal skin pH, whereas those in the acne group were much more likely to have a higher-than-normal pH.[64]

	% with Normal pH (men = pH 4-5.5) (Women – pH 4.5-5.5)[65]	% with > Normal pH
Control (Healthy Skin)	93%	6%
Acne Group	22%	77.5%

Cutibacterium acnes (previously known as Propionibacterium acnes) is a skin commensal (friendly bacteria) known to be associated with acne. It prefers a pH of 6-6.5 and has markedly reduced growth at lower pH.[66] One study revealed that the use of alkaline soap versus acidic products affected the number of outbreaks. The alkaline-soap-using group had an increase in the number of lesions while the acidic group had a reduction.[67]

Reducing skin pH reduces the inflammatory (Th2) response, and there is evidence that topical antibiotics, such as erythromycin, reduce skin pH, which may help explain their short-term effectiveness.[68, 69]

---

[62] Ali & Yosipovitch, 2013

[63] Prakash et al., 2017

[64] Prakash et al., 2017

[65] Kim et al., 2009

[66] Eo et al., 2016

[67] Eo et al., 2016

[68] Prakash et al., 2017

[69] Korting et al., 1993

As you can see, the skin's pH plays a vital role in its overall health and in the role of acne. In Part II of this book, I show you ways to optimise your skin's pH.

The Skin Microbiome

Your skin functions as the exterior interface between the human body and the environment, acting as a physical barrier to prevent the invasion of foreign microbes while providing a home for the commensal microbiota.

> *Commensal[70] = organisms in which one obtains food or other benefits from the other without damaging or benefiting it.*
>
> *Microbiota[71] = the microscopic organisms of a particular environment.*

The harsh physical landscape of skin, particularly the dry, nutrient-poor, acidic environment, also contributes to the adversity pathogens face when colonizing human skin. Despite this, the skin is colonised by a diverse microbiota.[72]

Our skin is completely coated in microbes. There are approximately 1,000,000 bacteria composed of hundreds of species on every square centimetre of our bodies.[73] Our skin is home to millions of bacteria, fungi and viruses that compose the skin microbiota.

Skin microorganisms have essential roles in the following:

- the protection against invading pathogens,
- the education of our immune systems and
- the breakdown of natural products like the microbes of the gut.

---

[70] 'Commensal,' n.d.

[71] 'Microbiota,' n.d.

[72] Byrd et al., 2018

[73] Finlay & Finlay, 2019

Pathogen:[74] a specific causative agent (such as a bacterium or virus) of disease.

As the largest organ in the human body, the skin is colonised by beneficial micro-organisms, but when the barrier is broken or the balance between commensals and pathogens is disturbed, skin disease—or even systemic disease—can result.

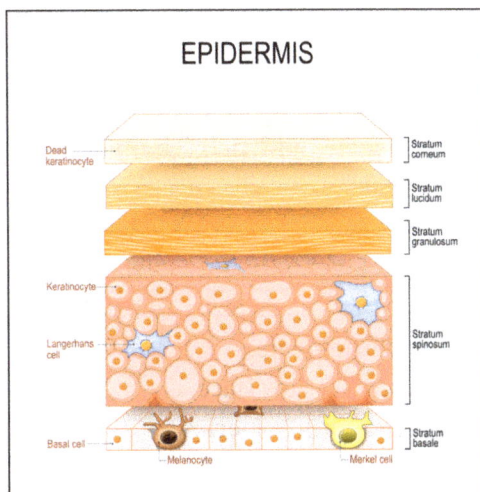

Studying the composition of the microbiota at different sites may be valuable for finding the cause of most skin disorders, such as acne, as well as eczema, dermatitis or psoriasis.

Structurally, the skin is composed of two distinct layers, the epidermis and the dermis. The outermost (the epidermis) is composed of layers of differentiated keratinocytes.

The top layer of the epidermis—or stratum corneum—is composed of terminally differentiated enucleated keratinocytes (also known as squames) that are chemically cross-linked to fortify the barrier of the skin.[75]

Keratinocyte:[76] a cell of the epidermis that produces keratin.

---

[74] 'Pathogen,' n.d.

[75] Segre, 2006

[76] 'Keratinocyte,' n.d.

Sweat glands are important for the maintenance of body temperature through the evaporation of water, which also acidifies the skin, making conditions unfavourable for the growth and colonisation of certain microorganisms.[77]

Sweat contains antimicrobial molecules, such as free fatty acids and antimicrobial peptides, that inhibit microbial colonization.[78]

Connected to the hair follicle and denser in oily sites, the sebaceous glands secrete lipid-rich sebum, a hydrophobic coating that lubricates and provides an antibacterial shield for hair and skin.[79]

The type of microbial communities on the skin is dependent on the physiology of the skin site, with changes in the relative abundance of the types of bacteria associated with moist, dry and sebaceous microenvironments.

Sebaceous sites (face, chest and back) are dominated by lipophilic *Propionibacterium* species.

> **Lipophilic:**[80] *having an affinity for lipids (such as fats)*

Bacteria that thrive in humid environments, such as the *Staphylococcus* and *Corynebacterium* species, were more abundant in moist areas, including the bends of the elbows and the feet. Fungal community composition is similar across core body sites, regardless of physiology.

So, if you have ever wondered—as did I—why you only tend to get acne on the face, chest and back and not the arms, legs or lower torso, it is likely because the face, chest and back are sebaceous sites dominated by the acne-related Propionibacterium species of bacteria (Cutibacterium acnes are members member of the Propionibacterium species).

---

[77] Grice & Segre, 2011

[78] Vieth & Sloan, 1986

[79] Byrd et al., 2018

[80] 'Lipophilic,' n.d.

Fungi of the genus *Malassezia* predominate on the core body and arms, whereas foot sites are colonised by a more diverse combination of *Malassezia* spp., *Aspergillus* spp., *Cryptococcus* spp., *Rhodotorula* spp., *Epicoccum* spp. and others.[81]

Compared to the intestines, the skin lacks many nutrients beyond basic proteins and lipids. To survive in such a cool, acidic and dry environment, our skin's resident microbiota has adapted to utilise resources present in sweat, sebum and the stratum corneum.

C. acnes, for example, can thrive in the anoxic sebaceous gland, using proteases to liberate the amino acid arginine from skin proteins and lipases to degrade triglyceride lipids in sebum. This releases free fatty acids, which promote bacterial adherence. Sebum levels on the cheek are abundant with *Propionibacterium* species.

Anoxic:[82] greatly deficient in oxygen.

Malassezia Species of Fungi (Fungal Acne)

The *Malassezia* species of fungi is the most abundant fungal organism on the skin. It co-exists with *C. acnes* and other bacteria.

Malassezia is the fungus thought to cause fungal acne.[83]

One study showed acne lesions were significantly reduced after administration of antifungal drugs. The authors suggested that *Malassezia* and not *C. acnes* was potentially the cause of acne not responding to treatment.[84]

The findings from several other studies are in support of this hypothesis. One study reported that *Malassezia restricta* and *Malassezia globosa* can be isolated from young acne patients.[85, 86]

---

[81] Takayasu, et al., 1980

[82] 'Anoxic,' n.d.

[83] Akaza et al., 2016

[84] Hu et al., 2010

[85] Song et al., 2011

[86] Numata et al., 2014

Another study showed the lipase (enzyme) activity of *Malassezia* is ~100 times higher than that of *P. acnes*.[87]

Malassezia can also hydrolyse triglycerides in the sebum to produce free fatty acids, which may affect the abnormal keratinisation of hair follicular ducts, chemotise polymorphonuclear neutrophils,[88, 89] and promote the secretion of pro-inflammatory cytokines from keratino-cytes and monocytes.[90, 91] Simply put, *Malassezia* can increase fatty acid production, increase skin cell development in the hair follicles poten-tially leading to a blockage and increase inflammation via activation of an immune response. It is the immune response that causes the acne lesions' redness.

How much *Malassezia* levels are affected on the skin via the gut-skin axis is unclear, but it is not beyond the scope of possibility that a *Malas-sezia* over-growth in the gut may be capable of relocating from the gut to the skin via the gut-skin axis. It is, therefore, important to optimise your gut microbiome (which is discussed in Chapter 6), whether you have bacterial or fungal acne.

The Gut-Skin Axis

Chronic skin conditions such as acne are complex and affected by many factors. Current evidence offers insight into how the skin and gut microbiome are connected. There is evidence the gut microbiome influ-ences other organ systems, and it has a particularly complex connection to the skin.[92]

Commensal—or friendly—bacteria in the gut help modulate sys-temic immunity and reduce inflammation, which has an impact on skin

---

[87] Akaza et al., 2012

[88] Katsuda et al., 2005

[89] Webster, 1995

[90] Kesavan et al., 1998

[91] Akaza et al., 2012

[92] Salem et al., 2018

health.[93] For example, short-chain fatty acids (SCFAs) are produced by commensal gut microbes when they ferment dietary fibre. SCFAs regulate the lifecycle of immune cells and have a protective role against the development of inflammatory disorders. This is relevant as acne has an inflammatory component.[94]

Another SCFA, butyrate, can positively modulate the activity of inflammatory cells such as cytokines and suppress inflammatory immune responses, and therefore, acne.[95]

Under certain conditions, commensal bacteria can undergrow, and pathogenic bacteria (and other microbes) can thrive. This creates dysbiosis (an imbalance in the amounts and types of bacteria) in the gut, which can have a negative impact on your health. Chemicals produced by these gut microbes may enter the bloodstream, build up in the skin, and impair skin health.[96] This may occur due to increased gut permeability, otherwise known as leaky gut syndrome.

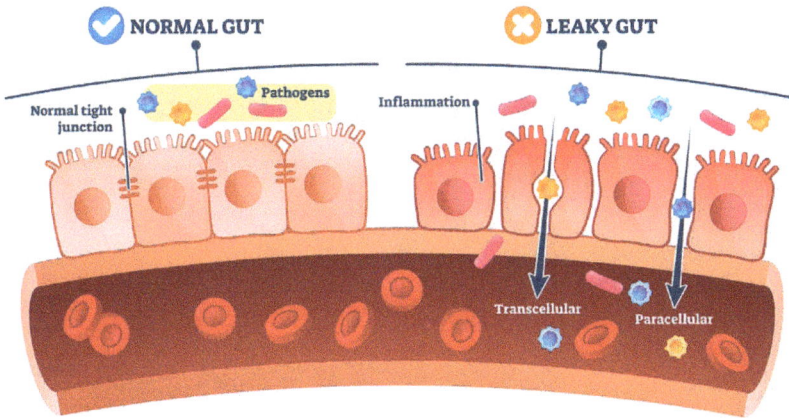

LEAKY GUT

NORMAL GUT · LEAKY GUT

Normal tight junction · Pathogens · Inflammation · Transcellular · Paracellular

---

[93] O'Neill et al., 2016

[94] O'Neill et al., 2016

[95] O'Neill et al., 2016

[96] O'Neill et al., 2016

If you have a healthy, diverse gut microbiome, it greatly increases—if not ensures—your health. Research has suggested a dysbiotic gut microbiome leads to disease and may be associated with skin disorders.[97, 98]

Rather than addressing the skin alone, it's crucial to consider the role of the gut microbiome in skin conditions, including acne.

There is evidence that acne is an inflammatory disease, and gut health may play a role in its development.[99, 100] Low levels of stomach acid are often associated with acne, and a more alkaline gastric pH enables bacteria from the colon to access the small intestine. This can cause gut dysbiosis, malabsorption of nutrients and small intestinal bacterial overgrowth (SIBO).[101]

Nutrient malabsorption may play a role in the development of acne as bacterial overgrowth competes with your cells for nutrients, impairing the absorption of nutrients. Studies have suggested the malabsorption of micronutrients—such as folate, chromium, selenium, omega-3 fatty acids and zinc—is associated with the development of acne.[102, 103]

The production of toxic metabolites resulting from SIBO can increase gut permeability (leaky gut syndrome), leading to systemic inflammation with an association with acne.[104, 105]

Factors associated with a modern Western lifestyle, such as antibiotic use, psychological and physical stress and diet, can adversely affect the gut microbiome, leading to gut dysbiosis and its downstream effects.[106]

----

[97] O'Neill et al., 2016

[98] Weiss & Katta, 2017

[99] Tanghetti, 2016

[100] Lee et al., 2019

[101] O'Neill et al., 2016

[102] O'Neill et al., 2016

[103] Lee et al., 2019

[104] Bures et al., 2010

[105] Bowe & Logan, 2011, p. 1

[106] Hawrelak & Myers, 2004

As I alluded to earlier, research has shown that antibiotic use can cause significant, unfavourable changes in the balance of commensal gut microbes, leading to increased susceptibility to pathogenic microbes in the gut, an overgrowth of fungi or *Clostridium difficile*, and reduced production of SCFAs.[107, 108, 109]

Stress also exerts unfavourable changes in the gut, including a decreased release of stomach acid and changes in gut motility (constipation and/or diarrhoea), creating an environment less favourable to the proliferation of beneficial bacteria.[110, 111, 112]

Psychological stress lowers mucin production (in the gut), decreases immunoglobulin A (IgA) production (IgA is a type of antibody) and causes a substantial and ongoing increase in stress hormones, all of which can lower defences against pathogenic microbes in the gut, allowing for their proliferation.[113, 114, 115] Therefore, reducing overall stress and having stress reduction behaviours in place—such as meditation, yoga, tai chi or qi gong—is strongly advised.

> *Mucins*[116] *are a family of proteins produced by epithelial tissues in most animals. Mucins' key characteristic is their ability to form gels; therefore, they are a key component in most gel-like secretions, serving functions from lubrication to cell signalling to forming chemical barriers.*

[107] Hawrelak & Myers, 2004

[108] Gorbach et al., 1988

[109] Gorbach, 1993

[110] Hawrelak & Myers, 2004

[111] Webster, 2005

[112] Zaenglein, 2016

[113] Hawrelak & Myers, 2004

[114] Melnik & Zouboulis, 2013

[115] Leo & Sivamani, 2014

[116] 'Mucin,' 2004

Dietary intake shapes the make-up and metabolic activities of gut microbes. Some diets promote the proliferation of beneficial microbes while other diets lead to unhealthy gut microbe activity.[117]

A varied diet maximises your nutrition and gut microbiome. Dietary restriction and the overuse of elimination diets can decrease gut microbe diversity and introduce you to potential nutrient deficiencies.[118, 119, 120]

In Part II of this book, I show you how to walk the tightrope of eliminating foods causing your acne and obtaining a varied diet to aid microbial diversity in your digestive system.

What Else Causes Acne?

Acne myths

Despite being one of the most widespread skin conditions, acne is also one of the most poorly understood. There are many myths and misconceptions about it:

'Acne is caused by a poor diet'

So far, research has not found any foods that cause acne. Eating a healthy, balanced diet is recommended because it's good for your heart and your health in general.

Above[121] is a section from the UK's National Health Service (NHS) website suggesting it is a myth that acne is caused by a poor diet, and research has not found **any** [my emphasis] foods causing acne.

---

[117] Hawrelak & Myers, 2004

[118] Zarogoulidis et al., 2014

[119] Li and Wang, 2014

[120] Soliman, 2013

[121] 'Overview: Acne,' 2017

I begin with this information because I want you to keep this in mind as you read through the rest of this section. It is further evidence of my earlier claims that the current medical paradigm does not believe diet is related to acne, and there is no research suggesting food can cause acne.

I invite you to review the medical establishment's belief after reading the evidence I am about to present to you.

Acne usually begins around the time of puberty. Adolescent males are more likely to have acne than females because of the effects of testosterone. Whilst most acne occurs in teenagers, 40-54% of men and women older than 25 years will have some degree of facial acne, and clinical facial acne persists into middle age in 12% of women and 3% of men.[122]

Genetic factors and/or propensities do play a role in acne. One study suggests that if both parents have acne, three out of four children will likely have acne, too. If one parent has acne, then one out of four of the children are also likely to have acne.[123] I would, however, add this does not prove a genetic propensity to acne as it may be the parents with acne taught their children the same behaviours or lived in the same environment causing their acne.

Many experts consider acne to be androgen-dependent, and an excess of androgen, either systemic or local (on the skin), is associated with more severe forms of the disease. Androgens control sebum secreted from the sebaceous gland and exacerbate the development of abnormal keratinisation by the follicular epithelium. This means androgens increase the production of greasy, sticky sebum and skin cells.

---

[122] Cordain et al., 2002

[123] Goulden et al., 1999

> 'Epithelium:[124] *a membranous cellular tissue that covers a free surface or lines a tube or cavity of an animal body and serves especially to enclose and protect the other parts of the body, to produce secretions and excretions, and to function in assimilation.'*

One research paper suggests endocrine (hormone) disorders producing excess androgens are important causal factors, which include:[125] (66)

- idiopathic adrenal androgen excess,
- partial defect in 21-hydroxylase and
- polycystic ovary syndrome.

If you have any of these conditions, it is likely they play a role in the cause of your acne.

According to research, free testosterone, dehydroepiandrosterone (DHEA), dehydroepiandrosterone sulphate (DHEA-S), and low sex-hormone-binding globulin (SHBG) levels have all been implicated in acne. Greater activity of the enzyme 5-α-reductase, which converts testosterone to the stronger androgen dihydrotestosterone (DHT), has been found in the skin of acne patients.[126, 127]

The increased 5-α-reductase activity is independent of systemic levels of androgens, which may explain the poor correlation between systemic levels of androgens and the severity of acne lesions.[128, 129]

Receptors for growth hormone and insulin-like growth factor (IGF-1) are present in the sebaceous gland. These hormones also stimulate sebum production. Conditions of growth hormone excess, such as acromegaly, are associated with increased sebum production and acne.

---

[124] 'Epithelium,' n.d.

[125] Pochi, 1982

[126] Pochi, 1982

[127] Darley et al., 1984

[128] Takayasu et al., 1980

[129] Sansone and Reisner, 1971

At high levels, insulin can also play a role by interacting with IGF-1 receptors, which promote the expression of enzymes responsible for androgen biosynthesis and conversion.[130]

Acromegaly:[131] *a disorder caused by excessive production of growth hormone by the pituitary gland and marked especially by progressive enlargement of hands, feet, and face.*

Exposure to industrial pollutants or certain medications can also increase the likelihood of acne, as well as everyday toxins, such as:

- mercury,
- cadmium and
- PCBs.

Polychlorinated biphenyl:[132] *any of several compounds that are produced by replacing hydrogen atoms in biphenyl with chlorine, have various industrial applications, and are toxic environmental pollutants which tend to accumulate in animal tissues. Called also* ***PCB.***

Medications and compounds that can cause acne lesions include:[133, 134]

- corticosteroids (used as anti-inflammatories),
- halogens (fluorine, chlorine, bromine, iodine, and astatine),
- isonicotinic acid (used in treating tuberculosis),
- diphenylhydantoin (used in treating epilepsy),

[130] Pochi, 1982

[131] 'Acromegaly,' n.d.

[132] 'Polychlorinated,' n.d.

[133] Webster, 2005

[134] Zaenglein et al., 2016

- lithium carbonate (used in the glass and ceramic industries and medicine, especially in the treatment of bipolar disorder),
- anabolic steroids (e.g., testosterone) and
- immunotherapeutic agents.

Lifestyle choices and exposures that can cause acne lesions include:[135, 136]

- machine oils,
- coal tar derivatives (used especially as industrial fuels, in making dyes, and in the topical treatment of skin disorders),
- chlorinated hydrocarbons (used as insecticides),
- cosmetics,
- pomades (a perfumed ointment; *especially* a fragrant hairdressing),
- over washing and
- repetitive rubbing.

It is for these reasons it is important to identify any toxins in your environment, and where possible, know how to safely remove toxins that have been stored in your cells. This is covered in chapters seven and eight.

The Big Four

Medical consensus suggests there are four major causes of acne:

1. **hyper-seborrhoea**—excess sebum production and changes in the sebum lipid profile;
2. **abnormal follicular keratinisation**—excess skin cell production;
3. *C. acnes* **proliferation in the pilosebaceous gland**; and
4. *inflammation* in response to the C. acnes proliferation.

---

[135] Webster, 2005
[136] Zaenglein et al., 2016

Around the time of puberty, increased androgen levels stimulate sebum production. This can change the lipid profile of the sebum itself (hyper-seborrhoea). The rise in androgens also increases the production of keratin by the cells lining the follicular canal.

> **Keratin:**[137] *basic proteins chiefly of epithelial cells and tissues that are relatively insoluble and resistant to degradation, form filaments which assemble into bundles to provide structural support and are the primary component of... the epidermal layer of skin.*

The formation of acne lesions begins in the upper portion of the follicular canal at the pore. The first microscopic change is increased keratinisation by the cells lining the follicular canal. Over time, this forms a follicular plug that blocks the canal and forms a comedone. Whether

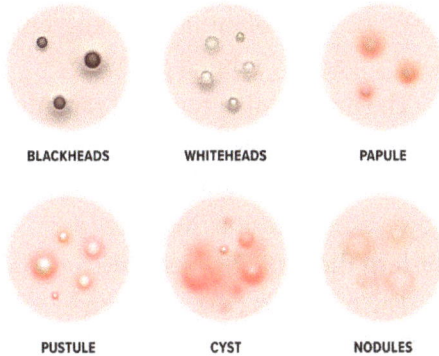

BLACKHEADS   WHITEHEADS   PAPULE

PUSTULE   CYST   NODULES

an open or closed comedone is formed depends on the degree of keratinisation and blockage of the duct. Open comedones (blackheads) form because blockages cause the sebum to move to the surface of the pore. The sebum oxidises to a black colour, giving the open comedone its characteristic colour.

When the duct is completely blocked, sebum becomes trapped beneath the surface, forming a closed comedone (whitehead). These events, in combination with inflammation caused by factors like physical irritation, diet, stress and cosmetics, can cause disruptions in the skin barrier.

---

[137] 'Keratin,' n.d.

Inflammation and a compromised skin barrier encourage the colonisation of the commensal bacteria *C. acnes,* which plays a key role in the formation and progress of acne lesions. The severity of acne lesions is thought to be determined by this complex interaction between hormones, keratinisation, sebum and bacteria.[138]

The mTOR Pathway and Acne

Another theory of the cause of acne is via the mTOR Pathway.

The aetiology of acne is multifactorial, including a wide array of genetic and environmental factors. It is a disease found primarily in Western societies that is completely absent in hunter-gatherer societies whose diets often include vegetables, meat and fruit and often lack dairy, sugar and refined grains.[139]

The mammalian target of rapamycin (mTOR) is a pathway that has shown a strong role in the pathogenesis of acne, and research shows a connection between a Western diet, mTOR and acne.

The mTOR is part of a complex pathway, often referred to as the PI3K/Akt/mTOR pathway, managing cellular energy and survival by monitoring both intra- and extra-cellular signals.

Phosphatidylinositol 3kinase (PI3K) and protein kinase B (Akt) are upstream modulators of mTOR, and together, all three create the PI3K/Akt/mTOR pathway.[140]

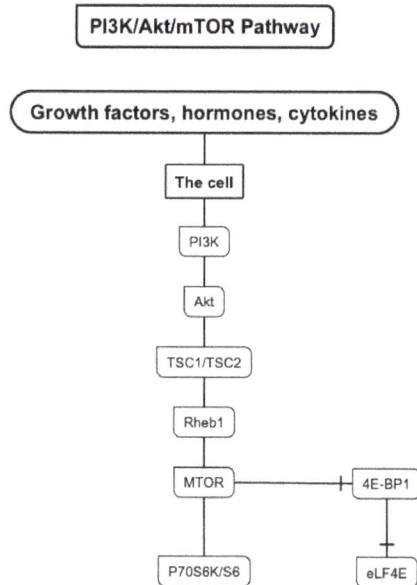

PI3K/Akt/mTOR Pathway

Growth factors, hormones, cytokines

The cell

PI3K

Akt

TSC1/TSC2

Rheb1

MTOR — 4E-BP1

P70S6K/S6   eLF4E

---

[138] Webster, 2005

[139] Melnick & Zouboulis, 2013

[140] Leo & Sivamani, 2014

The mTOR pathway includes two distinct multi-protein complexes: mTOR complex 1 (mTORC1) and mTOR complex 2 (mTORC2).

An important element in the pathway is Forkhead box transcription factor O1 (FoxO1), which inhibits the mTOR pathway when it is located in the nucleus but becomes inactive when exported into the cytosol.

> **'Cytosol:**[141] *the fluid portion of the cytoplasm exclusive of organelles and membranes. Called also ground substance.'*
> https://www.merriam-webster.com/dictionary/

PI3K/Akt/mTOR, along with FoxO1, all work together to monitor the nutritional status of the cell and to regulate a wide range of biological functions in the cell, including:[142, 143, 144, 145]

- cell growth,
- cell proliferation,
- cell survival,
- cell metabolism,
- cell cycle progression,
- gene transcription and
- protein synthesis.

mTOR complex 1

Metabolic homeostasis is, in large part, regulated by the cellular sensing of nutrients. An abundance or lack of nutrients either signals the cell to grow or conserve resources. mTORC1 is rapamycin-sensitive and

---

[141] 'Cytosol,' n.d.

[142] Leo & Sivamani, 2014

[143] Zarogoulidis et al., 2014

[144] Li & Wang, 2014

[145] Soliman, 2013

a main driver of cell growth by upregulating anabolic processes and downregulating catabolic processes.[146]

Increased activation of mTORC1 has been associated with a wide variety of diseases and conditions, including cancer, diabetes, insulin resistance, obesity, melanoma and acne.[147]

mTOR exists in at least two distinct protein complexes

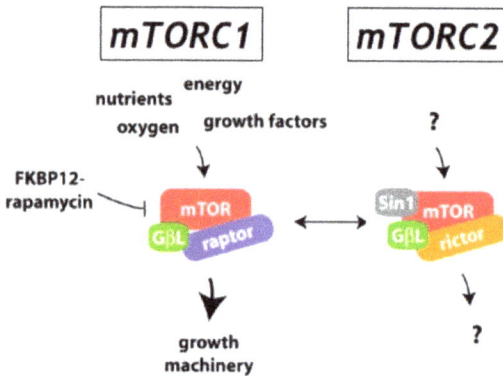

mTOR complex 2

mTORC2 is also involved in cellular growth and metabolism; however, it is rapamycin-insensitive and far less is known about it than mTORC1.[148, 149] It is involved in cell polarity and the organisation of the cytoskeleton in the cell, but the precise mechanism is still unknown.[150, 151]

---

[146] LaPlante & Sabatini, 2009

[147] Melnik, 2018

[148] Dgotto, 2006

[149] Monfrecola et al., 2016

[150] LaPlante & Sabatini, 2009

[151] Monfrecola et al., 2016

Functions of the mTOR pathway[152, 153, 154]

mTORC1	mTORC2
Cell growth	Cell growth
Cell metabolism	Cell metabolism
Lipid synthesis	Cell polarity
Lipid metabolism	Cytoskeletal regulation
Protein synthesis	
Autophagy	
Mitochondrial metabolism	
Mitochondrial biogenesis	
Microtubule organisation	

FoxO1: an mTORC1 Inhibitor

FoxO1 is a transcription factor involved in metabolism regulation found in all mammalian tissue.[155] It modulates the expression of genes across a wide array of functions, including glucose and lipid metabolism, cell differentiation, inflammation, and DNA damage repair.[156] FoxO1 is active in the cell's nucleus but can be inhibited when exported into the cell's cytoplasm.

In the nucleus, FoxO1 actively inhibits cell growth and metabolism; however, when it is extruded into the cytosol due to high nutrient sensing in the cell, it is effectively inactivated, so the cell enters an anabolic state.

---

[152] Soliman, 2013

[153] LaPlante & Sabatini, 2009

[154] Monfrecola et al., 2016

[155] Leo & Sivamani, 2014

[156] Leo & Sivamani, 2014

Both IGF-1 and insulin have been shown to inhibit nuclear FoxO1 levels. In the nucleus, FoxO1 performs the following functions:[157, 158]

- inhibits hepatic (liver) IGF-1 synthesis,
- inhibits lipogenesis via transcription factor SREPB-1c,
- inhibits protein synthesis,
- Inhibits androgen signalling
- inhibits T-cell activation and IL-1 activity,
- enhances antimicrobial peptide synthesis and
- reduces oxidative stress.

Put into simple terms, Fox01 in the nucleus of a cell reduces the likelihood of acne, and when outside the nucleus in the cell's cytosol increases the likelihood of acne as it allows an anabolic (growth) state and triggers an immune response and inflammation.

IGF-1 and insulin inhibit nuclear Fox01 levels, and therefore, increase the likelihood of acne. You'll soon find out why IGF-1 and insulin are so important!

What Activates the mTOR pathway?

The mTOR pathway is activated in response to many endogenous signals, such as hormones and growth factors, and exogenous factors, such as nutrients. mTORC1 drives cell growth and is influenced by several main signals, including growth factors, amino acids, lipids, energy status, inflammation and oxygen.[159, 160]

Growth factors activate mTOR through a variety of signals beginning with the binding of insulin and insulin-like growth factor-1

---

[157] Leo & Sivamani, 2014

[158] Melnik, 2015

[159] Soliman, 2013

[160] LaPlante & Sabatini, 2009

(IGF-1) to surface receptors on the cell.[161] High levels of insulin and IGF-1 can activate Akt, which can phosphorylate FoxO1 and lead to the exportation of FoxO1 into the cytosol.

> **Phosphorylate:**[162] *to cause (an organic compound) to take up or combine with phosphoric acid.*
> https://www.merriam-webster.com/dictionary/

Research has shown that people with acne have a greater expression of FoxO1 in the cytoplasm versus in the nucleus.[163]

Elevated insulin and IGF-1 can upregulate androgen receptor expression.[164] IGF-1 levels have been correlated with the physical manifestation of acne, and they are important to the pathogenesis of acne. Interestingly, people with Laron syndrome, a condition of the congenital deficiency of IGF-1, never develop acne unless treated with recombinant IGF-1.[165]

Other growth factors shown to promote mTOR include epidermal growth factor (EGF) and fibroblast growth factor (FGF).[166]

Amino acids leucine and glutamine play pivotal roles in mTORC1 activation. Leucine, an essential amino acid, is necessary for the activation of mTORC1 and is imported into the cell via glutamine transporters.[167, 168]

---

[161] LaPlante & Sabatini, 2009

[162] 'Phosphorylate,' n.d.

[163] Ju et al., 2017

[164] Melnik, 2012

[165] Melnik & Schmitz, 2013

[166] Soliman, 2013

[167] LaPlante & Sabatini, 2009

[168] 'High milk-/dairy intake High glycemic load image from Ju et al., 2017

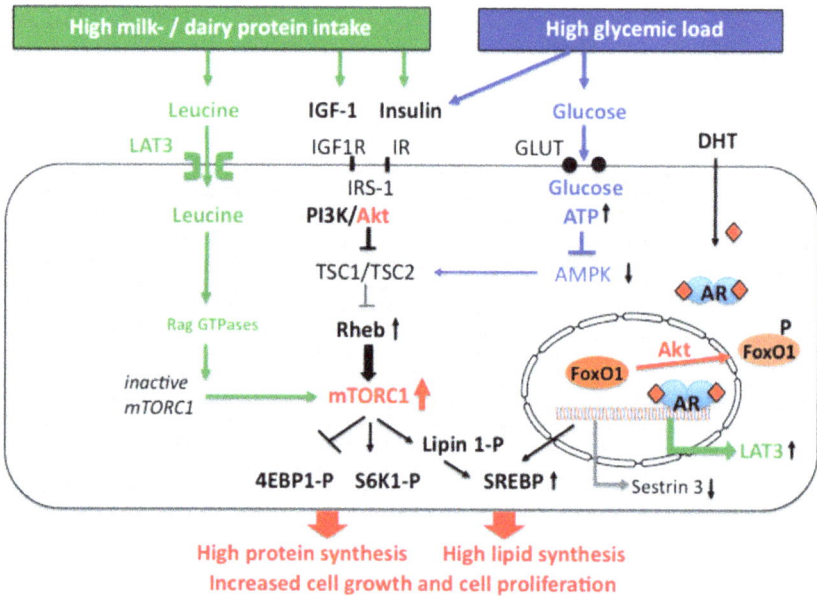

High protein synthesis   High lipid synthesis
Increased cell growth and cell proliferation

In addition to promoting the cellular uptake of leucine, glutamine is also involved in the growth of sebocytes and the production of lipids.[169]

In addition to leucine, other branched-chain amino acids, such as isoleucine and valine, have also been found to increase mTORC1.[170]

Palmitate, a saturated fatty acid, was shown to activate mTORC1.

Trans-fats resemble the chemical structure of palmitate, and while studies on their specific impact on mTORC1 remain to be done, they have been found to increase acne.[171]

Oleic acid has also been shown to stimulate mTORC1 and mTORC2, while omega-3 fatty acids have the opposite effect and were shown to inhibit mTORC1 activation.[172, 173]

---

[169] Melnik & Schmitz, 2013
[170] Monfrecola et al., 2016
[171] Melnik & Schmitz, 2013
[172] Melnik & Schmitz, 2013
[173] Menon et al., 2017

Energy Status, Inflammation & Oxygen Status

Energy status:

- AMP-activated protein kinase (AMPK) is a sensor of intracellular energy that transmits information about the energy status of a cell to mTORC1. When ATP levels are low, AMPK down-regulates the mTOR pathway.[174]

Inflammation:

- Pro-inflammatory cytokines (TNF-α and IL-1), send signals activating mTORC1, and researchers are starting to link this process to diseases such as tumour formation and insulin resistance.[175]

Oxygen status:

- When cells are low on oxygen, the resulting hypoxia generates multiple signals that down-regulate mTORC1.[176]

Signals Activating mTORC1[177, 178, 179, 180, 181, 182]

Signal	Examples
Energy	Glucose, ATP/ADP
Oxygen	O_2
Amino acids	Leucine, isoleucine, valine, glutamine

---

[174] LaPlante & Sabatini, 2009
[175] LaPlante & Sabatini, 2009
[176] LaPlante & Sabatini, 2009
[177] Li & Wang, 2014
[178] Soliman, 2013
[179] LaPlante & Sabatini, 2009
[180] Monfrecola et al., 2016
[181] Melnik, 2012
[182] Menon et al., 2017

Lipids	Saturated fats (palmitate, oleic acid), trans-fats
Inflammation	TNF-α, NF-κβ, IL-1α, IL-1β, IL-2, IL-4, IL-8, IL-12, Th1, Th17
Growth factors	Insulin, IGF-1, EGF, FGF

How Does mTOR Relate to Acne?

The mTOR pathway is involved in the critical growth and survival functions of the cell and is a necessary component of a healthy system. However, overactivation of the pathway can result in inflammation and acne. Researchers in Italy measured the skin of ten acne patients and ten controls to measure mTOR expression and found that mTOR was significantly elevated in the skin of acne patients.[183]

The lesioned skin of acne patients had a 20.77-fold increase in mTOR gene expression versus controls, and non-lesioned skin showed a 17.96-fold increase.[184]

Humans must go through physiologically appropriate periods of high growth both as babies and during puberty, and these processes are driven by an increase in insulin and IGF-1, both of which upregulate mTORC1.[185, 186]

Puberty is also a time of increased hormone production in adolescents, including testosterone. IGF-1 stimulates both the production of androgens as well as the conversion of testosterone to dihydrotestosterone (DHT), which is ten times more active than testosterone.[187] Acne is a skin disorder afflicting over 85% of adolescents, and it is this increased production of IGF-1 and testosterone that creates a fertile ground for the pathogenesis of acne.[188]

---

[183] Monfrecola et al., 2016

[184] Monfrecola et al., 2016

[185] Leo & Sivamani, 2014

[186] Melnik, 2012

[187] Leo & Sivamani, 2014

[188] Leo & Sivamani, 2014

The sebaceous gland's function is to produce and secrete sebum that lubricates and augments the skin's barrier. A normal physiologic rise in sebum production occurs from the ages of around nine to 17 years old, corresponding to puberty.[189] However, in acne, there is enhanced activity of the glands as they produce an excess of sebum with an altered lipid composition.[190]

The increased IGF-1 in puberty is a part of this process, and it promotes growth via sebaceous gland proliferation and lipogenesis (including sebum production).[191] In people with acne, the PI3K/Akt/mTOR pathway is upregulated, increasing lipogenesis (lipid production) in sebocytes and preventing cell death, so you end up with an increased number of skin cells.[192]

mTORC1 specifically stimulates transcription factor sterol regulatory element binding protein 1 (SREBP1), which increases the production of sebum in the sebaceous gland.[193]

Androgens and the regulation of androgen receptors are key drivers of acne pathogenesis, and the role of the mTOR pathway in regulating the interplay between androgens, androgen receptors, and insulin/IGF-1 has been clearly demonstrated.[194] The sebaceous gland is the part of skin most active in synthesising steroids.[195]

Androgens contribute to acne by upregulating sebum gland growth and production and through increasing inflammation.[196, 197]

---

[189] Bhat et al., 2017

[190] Bhat et al., 2017

[191] Leo & Sivamani, 2014

[192] Melnik, 2017

[193] Monfrecola et al., 2016

[194] Ju et al., 2017

[195] Ju et al., 2017

[196] Ju et al., 2017

[197] Bhat et al., 2017

DHT is also shown to upregulate SREBP-1, and when combined with an increased IGF-1, SREBP-1 expression during puberty can result in the overproduction of sebum.[198]

The occurrence of acne in traditional hunter-gatherer populations has not been documented despite its prevalence in Western society as a normal feature of puberty. Therefore, we cannot say that acne is a normal physiological process of human adolescence. However, when these same hunter-gatherers move to urban areas and adopt a Western-style diet, they often develop acne.[199]

Over the past several years, research has shown a clear link between a Western diet and the pathogenesis of acne.[200] Western diets are full of sugar and refined carbohydrates that have a high glycaemic load and can cause chronic low-grade hyperinsulinemia (high levels in insulin), which are shown to impair FoxO1 function.[201, 202]

Dairy protein, a high glycaemic load and lipids can all increase insulin and IGF-1, thereby exacerbating acne.[203, 204]

Research has shown the bioactivity of free serum androgens and free serum IGF-1 is regulated by the glycaemic load of the diet, with a higher glycaemic load upregulating both. Refined carbohydrates and sugar contribute to a high glycaemic load. Researchers in Turkey tested 50 patients with acne against 36 control subjects and found that dietary glycaemic index and dietary glycaemic load levels were significantly higher in acne patients.[205]

[198] Ju et al., 2017

[199] Monfrecola et al., 2016

[200] Monfrecola et al., 2016

[201] Leo & Sivamani, 2014

[202] Danby, 2013

[203] Leo & Sivamani, 2014

[204] Monfrecola et al., 2016

[205] Çerman, 2016

Conversely, a low glycaemic diet has been shown to positively impact acne by downregulating androgens and IGF-1, thereby decreasing inflammation and reducing the size of sebaceous glands.[206, 207]

The purpose of milk is to facilitate the rapid growth of baby mammals, containing IGF-1, androgens, and amino acids. IGF-1 is found in milk, but milk also triggers the production of endogenous IGF-1 in mammals.[208, 209] In both adults and children, the consumption of milk raises serum IGF-1 levels and has been linked to hyperinsulinemia and insulin resistance.[210] Milk also contains androgens that activate mTORC1 and inhibit FoxO1, leading to a proliferation of keratinocyte production and an increase in sebum production.[211]

Milk has been shown to aid insulin in exposing androgen receptors, making a person more susceptible to circulating androgens. Dairy is also rich in leucine, glutamine and palmitic acid, all drivers of the mTOR pathway, as previously noted. Leucine is found in both meat and dairy products, and palmitic acid is found in butter and cream.[212]

Dairy is one of the highest sources of leucine, with whey protein containing 14% leucine, whereas beef contains only 8%.[213] Milk also contains approximately twice the amount of glutamine per 100

---

[206] Melnik, 2012

[207] Melnik & Schmitz, 2013

[208] Melnik, 2012

[209] Danby, 2013

[210] Melnik, 2012

[211] Danby, 2013

[212] Melnik & Schmitz, 2013

[213] Melnik & Schmitz, 2013

g serving as beef, with 8.09 g of glutamine in milk versus only 4.74 g in beef.[214]

As noted previously, lipids can also activate mTOR. Therefore, it is unsurprising that the consumption of increased saturated fat in the diet aggravated acne in several studies.[215] I would add to this that it might not be fats in the meat, per se. If the meat is not of high quality, it is likely the fat of the meat is toxic, as mammals store toxins in their fat cells.

Food Suggested by Research to Have a Causal Link to Acne:

When looking at most of the research on diet and acne, a few items seem to appear quite regularly in the literature. As we have seen above, the following nutrients are known to stimulate the mTOR pathway:

- glucose,
- amino acids leucine, glutamine, isoleucine and valine and
- fats such as trans fatty acids, palmitate, and oleic acid.

This would suggest that food such as bread, fruit, sugar, cakes, biscuits/cookies, ice cream, sweets/candy, soft drinks, dairy products, milk, butter, cream, meat, olive oil and nuts (especially peanuts and walnuts) could potentially be causing your acne via stimulation of the mTOR pathway.

Knowing that research has identified these foods as being potentially causative of acne, does it not make you wonder how the UK's National Health Service can still suggest that 'so far research has not found any foods that cause acne'?

Could it be there is a conflict of interest somewhere in the system that doesn't want to see a reduction in profits for acne products? I'll let you make that decision on your own.

---

[214] Melnik & Schmitz, 2013

[215] Melnik & Schmitz, 2013

Nutrients that Help to Block the mTOR Pathway

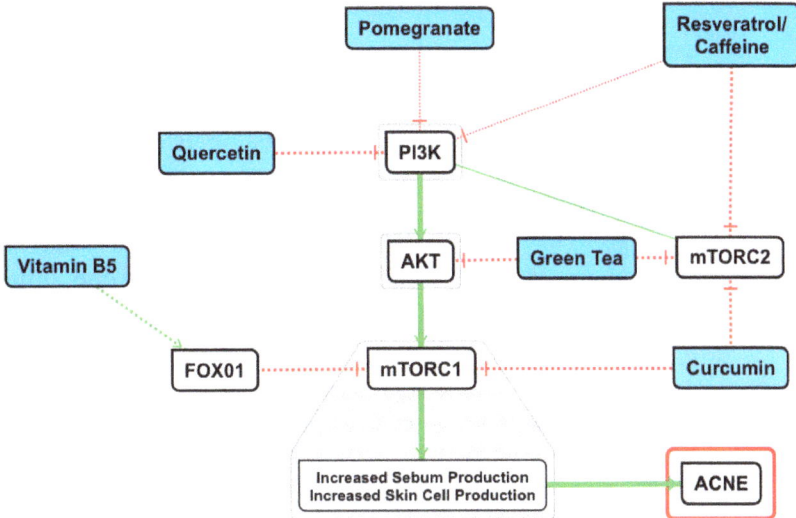

According to Dr Julie Greenberg[216] from The Centre for Integrative Dermatology in Los Angeles, California, a number of fibre-rich foods help to block the mTOR pathway, including a number of vegetables, preferably all the colours of the rainbow, plus:

- pomegranate,
- quercetin,
- vitamin B5,
- resveratrol,
- caffeine (not recommended),
- green tea and
- curcumin.

---

[216] Image adapted from Greenberg (2021).

Chapter summary/Key takeaways

In summary:

- Current medical advice suggests there is no research linking diet and acne, despite the prevalence of evidence.

- The pH of skin is crucial. The ideal, healthy pH of skin is 4-6, a slightly acidic environment. C. acnes prefer a more alkaline environment, with a pH of around 6-6.5. Acne sufferers have been shown to have a higher skin pH compared to non-sufferers.

- There are approximately 1,000,000 bacteria composed of hundreds of species on every square centimetre of our bodies. Different bacteria tend to colonise in separate regions of the skin. C. acnes tend to colonise in sebaceous sites, such as the face, chest and back.

- *Malassezia* species also seem causative of fungal acne in some people. *Malassezia* has been shown to increase free fatty acids in the sebum, which may affect the abnormal keratinisation of hair follicular ducts and increase pro-inflammatory cytokines on the skin.

- Gut health has been shown to play a role in acne via gut hyperpermeability, nutrient malabsorption, gut dysbiosis and the production of toxic metabolites.

- Excess androgens, industrial pollutants, medications and lifestyle choices have been shown to cause acne.

- There are four medical consensus causes of acne: hyper-seborrhoea, abnormal follicular keratinisation, C. acnes proliferation and inflammation. However, other research suggests there are more than these four factors.

- The mammalian target of rapamycin (mTOR) is a pathway shown to have a strong role in the pathogenesis of acne, and research is showing a connection between a Western diet, mTOR and acne.

- Nutrients known to stimulate the mTOR pathway include glucose; the amino acids leucine, glutamine, isoleucine and valine; and fats such as trans fatty acids, palmitate, and oleic acid. This suggests that many foods in the Western diet could cause acne in those who are genetically susceptible despite the medical establishment's denials.

Part II of the book explains your roadmap to clear skin.

PART II

YOUR ROADMAP TO
CLEAR SKIN

CHAPTER 3

SETTING YOUR MINDSET FOR SUCCESS

● ●

'A man becomes what he thinks about all day long.'

Ralph Waldo Emerson

Having coached clients for well over a quarter of a century, I can tell you that even when people know exactly what they need to do to be successful, if they are not in the right mindset, they will not do what is needed to be successful.

Whatever you do, do not consider skipping this chapter. Skipping this chapter could be the quickest route to failure.

I can teach you the best system to overcome acne, but if you don't follow through with it, is it going to work? Obviously not.

My psychic powers have kicked in, and I can hear you say, 'But of course, I'm going to follow through; I really want to get rid of my acne, once and for all.'

My experience of helping hundreds of clients over the years has shown that the path to success is never a straight one on its way to the summit. It is often a road with bumps along the way. That's life, and I want you to be ready to properly react when you encounter those bumps.

Too many times, I have seen people give up at the first challenge they come across. Sometimes, they don't see results as quickly as they would like and get frustrated or lose motivation. I want you to remember that there will be challenges along the way. You might take one step forwards and two steps backwards at times; that is life. But I want you to be ready to respond. As Stephen Covey, author of *The 7 Habits of Highly Effective People*, said, the 'ability to respond' is to have 'responsibility'.

Whilst I can help you along the way, I can't do the day-to-day tasks for you. In the following chapters, I teach you what you will need to succeed, but the responsibility is on you to follow through with the advice. I want you to feel empowered to take on these lifestyle changes so you can live the rest of your life without having to worry about what your skin looks like, just as I have for over two decades.

In this chapter, we cover:

- how the phrase, 'you are what you think' applies,
- goal setting,
- setting core values and
- planning to overcome obstacles before they arise.

You Are What You Think

Our thoughts can work for us or work against us. They can enhance our lives if we think positively, or they can make our lives more challenging if we think with fear, dread and negativity. We greatly benefit when we oversee our minds and only allow thoughts enhancing our wellbeing to make us feel more harmonious with everything around us. Every thought we have, and every word we speak has internal and external consequences. If you want clear skin, you cannot dwell on how your skin is right now and how bad it makes you feel.

I'm sure you've heard of the placebo effect. It is often discussed during medical research studies in which medications are tested against placebos, which are often sugar pills or saline injections, to assess whether a medication is safe and effective compared to the placebo (in other words, no medication at all).

We often see that people's health improves even when they have taken a placebo and there is no physiological reason why they should have got better. The improvement was caused by their thoughts and beliefs about the treatment they received. They believed they were receiving an effective treatment, and that alone was enough to create wellness.

So, a 'placebo effect' is when someone thinks or believes they are going to get better, and they do. One example includes a family member of mine who suffers from severe hay fever. Their doctor gave them an inhaler to use, as most of the oral medications hadn't worked. Very quickly, for the first time in years, their hay fever was gone. One day, this family member took their inhaler from the cupboard, opened their mouth, and pushed down on the button to release the gas into their mouth. Another family member approached and asked why they hadn't taken the cap off the inhaler to allow the gas to escape. It turns out they had never taken the cap off and hadn't received any of the medication, but did not experience the effects of hay fever. That's a great example of how the placebo effect works. Ironically, as soon as they started using the inhaler properly, the hay fever returned.

There is also the opposite of the placebo effect, called the 'nocebo effect'. This occurs when someone believes they are going to become ill or die, and they become ill or die. Examples of this are seen with cancer patients. Often, a patient is told by their oncologist that they have a certain amount of time to live, and the person dies within days of their prognosis. Is this because oncologists have psychic powers, or is it because most patients have complete—often blind—faith in doctors?

We also see terminal cancer patients who are told by their oncologists they have weeks or days to live yet survive for several decades afterwards. This could be, at least in part, because they didn't believe they were going to die despite having a 'diagnosis' of terminal cancer.

All of this goes to show that how you think can have a great effect on whether you overcome your acne. In fact, I would suggest it is the most important factor of success.

It is also worth bearing in mind that everything in the universe has a frequency. This means that everything vibrates, including whatever you are standing, sitting, or lying on. Solid things have a lower vibrational frequency, and as things become less solid, they vibrate (or resonate) at a higher frequency.

Take your mobile phone, for instance. You cannot see the radio frequency waves flowing in and out of the device because the radio waves—or microwaves—are vibrating too quickly for your visual receptors to see them. Also, you will be aware that dogs can hear higher frequencies than humans; the hearing receptors of dogs can pick up vibrations our human hearing system cannot.

There are subtle energy systems in the body, such as chakras and energy meridians, which the ancient Indians and Chinese were aware of thousands of years ago. How did they know they were there if we can't see them now? Could it be these ancient people were able to see different frequencies than we do now? Have modern lifestyles prevented us from seeing a wider range of frequencies?

What we do know is that these subtle energy systems exist, and they vibrate at a frequency too high for most people to see. Interestingly, some people can see them. They can also be picked up with Kirlian photography.

Where am I going with this, I hear you ask? Well, just like everything else in the universe, our thoughts are also vibrations. Electroencephalograms, for instance, are used to pick up brain waves, implying that the frequencies of our thoughts can be measured. This is well accepted in science—I haven't eaten too many wild mushrooms or smoked any exotic herbs and lost my mental faculties, in case you were wondering.

So, our thoughts have specific vibrations, and quantum physics tells us that like attracts like. Using the mind to create outcomes in life has worked for me and my clients for many years. This means that if you want great skin, you can begin to create it with your thoughts.

By thinking that you have great skin right now in the present tense, you are creating the vibration of great skin and making it more likely to happen and happen quicker. I'm not suggesting this is all you must do—you still need to do the physical work—but creating the vibration will make achieving great skin that much more likely.

What I do, and suggest my clients do, is create a positive affirmation statement around a specific goal. All of the words need to be positive words—no negative words (like no, not, without, etc.) are allowed. Once drafted, the positive affirmation statement is spoken out loud in the present tense many times each day to help create the vibration.

Some people are sceptical or critical of this technique, and it will not work for those who are because they are creating the wrong vibration. In my experience, it is very effective for those who use it properly, but you still need to do the physical work.

In the next section, you will begin setting your goals. Once you have set your goals, you can create a positive affirmation statement and begin using it immediately, several times per day. Call it a 'performance-enhancing vibration' if you'd like; only these performance-enhancers are perfectly legal.

Goal Setting

I am going to reiterate what I said in the previous section: DO NOT skip this part of the book. It is crucial for your success that your mind is in tip-top shape to take on the tasks you will learn in the following chapters. I really want you to take your time and not rush this section. Find a quiet space to do it where you will not be disturbed. Complete each question below carefully and as thoughtfully as you possibly can.

The Rules for Answering the Questions:

I do have a few rules for you when completing the answers in this section. You cannot use the following words:

- acne
- zits
- spots
- breakouts

- blemishes
- whiteheads
- blackheads
- itchy
- painful
- swelling
- bumpy
- flaky
- sore
- red

or any other term related to acne.

- not
- free-from
- less
- don't
- won't
- without or
- any 'negative' word.

Got that? Great. Let's begin.

Please answer the following questions as carefully and honestly as possible.

1. Close your eyes and imagine your skin is exactly how you want it to be right now (not how it is now). Please describe your skin in as many words as possible now that you have achieved your goal. To help, you might want to describe how your skin looks and feels. Can you hear anything? Can you smell anything? Can you taste

anything? Remember not to use any of the banned words listed above! Please write your goals in the box below:

[   ]

2. Based on what you answered in question 1, is your goal specific, or is it vague?

Specific/Vague?

Review your answer and ensure that it is specific.

3. Can you measure your goal?

For instance, how many days in a row would you need to experience clear skin for you to say you had achieved success? If you'd be happy with six months of clear skin or however you want your skin to be, then great. It could be one year, two years or ten years with completely clear skin. Only you can make these decisions, as they are your goals. What is it about your goal that can be measured? Please write your answer in the box below:

[   ]

4. Is your goal realistic and achievable?

Yes/No?

For most, the possibility of having clear skin is very realistic (as long as you are willing to do the work). However, as an example, if you have severe pitting and scarring, it might be unrealistic to think it can be reversed using the advice in this book. Being realistic is important when avoiding disappointment.

5. What is your time scale for achieving your goal?

This is crucial. Setting a date by which to achieve your goal should help you stay motivated and on track each day to do what you need to achieve your goal within your chosen deadline. If you know you have a big day coming up—such as a wedding, holiday, or big social event—that can be great, as the date is generally fixed and can't be changed. If you follow all the recommendations in this book and stay consistent in your daily tasks, then, for most, it should take no longer than 6-12 months (the quickest results I've seen are over two weeks). However, for some, if there is a lot of toxicity to deal with, it can take longer, and you shouldn't rush detoxing.

Date: _ _ /_ _ /_ _ _ _.

6. Now that you have set your goal, you can use it to set your positive affirmation statement in the present tense, which you will say out loud several times per day. I'll give you a helping hand here—remember: positive words only!

I am happy and grateful now that...

I have also provided you with access to online forms you can complete and either print out or upload to the smart device of your choice. You can find the form at https://eliminateadultacne.com// resources

Once you have completed all the questions on goal-setting, it is time to move to the next section to set your core values.

Setting Core Values

Core values drive our decision-making and behaviour and help form beliefs. They serve as criteria or standards, guiding the choices of our actions and their evaluation. We decide what is justified or not based on the possible impact our decisions have on our values.

To identify our personal core values, we ask ourselves questions like:

- What do I stand for and not stand for?
- What goals do I want to attain?
- What makes me happy?

In the book, *How to Eat, Move & Be Healthy,*[217] Paul Chek suggests determining your core values based on his 4 Doctor Coaching model. His 4 Doctors include:

- Dr Happiness
- Dr Quiet
- Dr Diet
- Dr Movement

[217] 2004

In Chek's model, he suggests using the following questions to help set your core values (please complete the following, which I have adapted from Chek's model):

Dr Happiness:

I am happy when I: _____

_____

_____

_____

Dr Quiet:

To feel at my best, I need _____ hours of sleep per night.

For optimal regeneration, I am in bed by _____ and wake at ____.

I devote ____ minutes daily to relaxing and calming my mind. My ideal time for inner practise each day is ____.

I honour rest days from work on which days of the week? _____

I honour rest days from exercise on which days of the week? _____

I create times for relaxation in the following ways: _____

_____

_____

Dr Diet:
I feel best when I eat for my individual needs and commit to following Dr Diet's values:

☐ eating organic produce and fresh foods
☐ eating food based on seasonal availability

- [ ] rotating food for a variety
- [ ] eating meals at regular times each day
- [ ] drinking 0.03 litres of water per kg of body weight per day (not tap water)
- [ ] using diet logging to individualise my food and drink needs, meal-to-meal
- [ ] avoiding food I know will exacerbate my acne

Dr Movement:

I feel best when I balance workouts with gentle forms of exercise:

Work out _____ x per week for how long? _____

Gentle exercise _____ x per week for how long? _____

(Gentle exercise includes slow movements, gentle forms of yoga, tai chi, qi gong and walking in nature)

Stretch my muscles for _____ minutes _____ days per week.

It's great that you have your first set of core values to help you make the right choices going forwards. Please bear in mind that if you start living a life outside of these core values, your chance of overcoming your acne once and for all will reduce. So, it is important that you stick to your core values.

As you go through the rest of the sections of this book and you begin to learn more about what you need to do to be successful, you may need to come back to this section on core values and repeat the process for optimal results. I also recommend you do this process on a yearly basis at an absolute minimum.

I have also provided you with access to an online form you can complete and either print out or upload to the smart device of your choice. You can find the form at https://eliminateadultacne.com//resources

Plan to Overcome Obstacles Before They Arise

I am sure you have heard the modern-day proverb widely attributed to Alan Lakein:

Failing to plan is planning to fail.

This is very true when it comes to the food you buy when you do your cooking or planning to eat out at a restaurant. What many people fail to do is plan for potential obstacles that might get in the way of their success.

Several things with which I have seen people derail their healthy lifestyle plans include:

- socialising with friends,
- watching or playing sports,
- dinner parties with family or friends,
- weddings,
- holidays/vacations,
- travelling (personal or business),
- shopping,
- business meetings at mealtimes (breakfast, lunch, or dinner),
- work canteens and restaurants,
- work parties,
- entertaining clients and
- conferences

I've heard this many times. People say situations come up like those listed above, meaning they were unable to stay on track. Without question, the above scenarios make things a little challenging, but unlike what most people think, you still have the ability to respond to the situation. If you wait until you arrive at the event or activity, then you might well be limited in your choices. However, if you plan ahead, the amount of control you have and the ability to stay on track will greatly increase.

One of the greatest excuses I hear is that when any of the above events occur, they do not have control over the food they can eat, but is that really true? What they are saying is, 'I do not have the ability to respond to the situation,' or 'I have not planned ahead and am left with minimal options.'

There are several things you can do to stay on track and maintain a level of control over the food you eat. Regardless of the event, you can always investigate ahead of time.

Here are some questions you may wish to consider:

Find out what is on the menu. This may require a phone call or a little Internet search. You can find out whether they serve organic food or have a gluten-free menu, for instance.

Do they prepare and cook their food properly or do they destroy their food in a microwave oven?

What drinks are available?

What restaurants are nearby if you are going to be out all day?

Many solutions for staying on track do require a little work, but if you are serious about having clear skin for the rest of your life, it is a very small price to pay.

Some successful solutions clients have used include:

- taking their own food from home (even on aeroplanes);
- completing a weekly meal plan;
- cooking on weekends and freezing ready-to-use meals during the week;
- taking a little food to add to what is available at the event;
- taking their own drinking water;
- choosing restaurants serving organic food that have gluten-free options;
- asking their workplace to provide healthier and gluten-free options;
- telling their work clients they are teetotal under doctor's orders;

- avoiding ingredients causing acne and insisting on gluten-free when overseas, where they can't access organic food that is right for their type;

- researching holiday destinations and visiting locations with a reputation for high-quality food;

- letting hosts of dinner parties or family meals know of your dietary requirements ahead of time and asking them to cater to you, bringing your own food with you if they are unable to (or unwilling) to do as you ask and

- inviting people to dinner with you so you will be in control of the menu.

It is important for you to write down all the situations (or events) that could be potential stumbling blocks to your success. You can use the list above for inspiration.

Next, list all the things you can do ahead of time to ensure you are ready to deal with any outcome and stay on track on the road to clear skin for the rest of your life.

Chapter summary/Key takeaways

In summary:

- Your mind has the power to make you well and the power to make you ill.

- Everything in the known universe has a vibration, including our thoughts. It is important that we create positive vibrations to attract positive outcomes.

- Positive affirmations can be used daily to help generate the right vibrations for attracting clear skin. These should be said out loud and frequently throughout the day and with a belief in what you say.

- It's important to set goals using positive words and set goals that are specific, measurable and achievable yet challenging and within a set timeframe.

- Core values drive our decision-making and behaviour and form beliefs.

- It is important to set your core values, so you will have an array of guiding behaviours you are willing to do to achieve clear skin every day for the rest of your life.

- Failing to plan is planning to fail. It is essential to plan ahead of time to ensure you are able to put everything you need to be successful into practice.

- Planning for future potential obstacles to your success is vital. Having a plan to overcome every potential eventuality will put you in a rock-solid position to be successful in your quest for life-long clear skin.

In the next chapter, you will learn about the Acne Elimination Diet.

SUCCESS STORY 1

Meet Amir.

Amir was a 42-year-old professional man suffering from acne. He was overweight, suffering from low confidence, and had very low energy levels when he first came to me. He was also spending £400 per month on products to cover up his acne.

His skin was very oily, his face and scalp were covered in acne, and he worried it might start to affect his work.

Amir was a sugar lover, and it took him some time to wean himself off of sugar. Slowly, over time, Amir made the necessary changes. Upon testing his gut microbiome, it was discovered that he did have a minor imbalance of gut microbes, including Staphylococcus Aureus, which is often linked to skin conditions. However, I have seen much, much worse gut results.

He had hormone imbalances, which would have affected his energy levels and a number of food sensitivities that may have also caused his acne.

He was a slow starter in terms of changing his diet and lifestyle, and his progress was initially slow to non-existent. Amir was also given supplementation to help rebalance his gut microbiome and hormones.

A few months into the programme, we had a little heart-to-heart, and I made it clear to him that unless he fully committed to the programme, he simply wasn't going to be successful. I half-expected Amir to throw in the towel at that point, but to my surprise, it was just the kick up the backside he needed.

He knuckled down and started eating right for his Metabolic Type®, finally started eliminating sugar from his diet (with a lot of perseverance), and within a few weeks, his skin improved to the point where he had clear skin for the first time in 30 years.

I believe the main things contributing to his success were cutting out the sugar and sensitive foods and the protocol for rebalancing his gut microbiome.

CHAPTER
4

THE ACNE ELIMINATION DIET

'Let food be thy medicine, and let medicine be thy food.'

Hippocrates

In this chapter, I show you the Acne Elimination Diet.
The Acne Elimination Diet is crucial if you want to achieve perfect, glowing skin and finally say goodbye to red, blotchy, itchy, painful, embarrassing and ugly skin. After all, you are what you eat! Or perhaps more importantly, you are what you digest.

I will say that if you have mercury fillings or root canal-filled teeth, it might be the most important thing to address. If you do have mercury fillings or root canal-filled teeth, please go to Chapter 8.

Whilst you are dealing with any fillings, please continue with all the other processes in this chapter.

Metabolic Typing®

Metabolic Typing® gives you the foundation for improving your health and therefore, your skin from the inside out.

Metabolic Typing® might be all you need to do to achieve clear skin and regain your self-esteem and confidence. It forms the foundation for the health of all the systems in your body, including all your organs, of which your skin is just one. It is, therefore, crucial that you follow a diet right for your Metabolic Type®, even if you use some of the other techniques in this book. Eating right for your Metabolic Type® is a non-negotiable option.

What you put in your mouth has a major effect on your whole body as well as your skin. Think about it: if you had a plant that was dying, you'd wonder what you had to feed it to make it better. You wouldn't, for instance, spray paint its leaves green because they were turning brown. Health and healthy skin come from the inside out.

If you put junk into your body, you'll get junk out. Every action in the universe has a consequence, which is sometimes known as cause and effect. Some people might get acne from inadequate nutrition, whilst others might be obese, have diabetes or heart disease or possibly develop cancer.

Quite simply, Metabolic Typing® is the ultimate diet if you want to detoxify and improve the look of your skin.

Metabolic Typing® understands that every one of us is unique. What is right for you is not necessarily good for your partner, friends, or work colleagues, so I am not going to spell out a specific Clear Skin Diet that everyone can follow because that is not how nature works.

William Wolcott, the world's most renowned expert on Metabolic Typing® and author of *The Metabolic Typing Diet,* has made it clear that the right diet for you is predominantly dependent on your genetics, and secondly, on your environment. At a basic level, if your ancestors over the last 10,000 years came from a cold climate where the ground freezes for a part of the year, and there was an abundance of game meat available, your body is likely to flourish with a diet high in animal-based foods plus a small amount of plant-based food.

Conversely, if your ancestors came from a warm climate with access to vegetation all year round and very little meat or fish available, your body is likely to flourish with a diet high in plant-based foods with a small amount of animal-based food.

Not only does eating right for your Metabolic Type® increase energy, normalise body weight and eliminate cravings, but it also enables optimal energy production in every cell of the body. When each cell in your body produces an adequate amount of energy, it optimises the detoxification of the cells. Optimal detoxification is a key aspect in helping prevent acne in the long run.

Metabolic Typing® also allows you to stabilise blood sugar levels, and therefore, insulin and IGF-1 hormone levels. Blood sugar can be tested using a glucometer you can buy online or via your local pharmacy. It is simple to do and requires a simple finger prick to test.

I have been a Certified Metabolic Typing® Advisor since 2004 and have helped many people achieve amazing health, including helping them (and myself) to achieve great skin. I highly recommend taking the Metabolic Typing® Questionnaire (for a small fee) to find your 'type' and establish the food that is perfect for you.

> You can find instructions to take the online questionnaire at
> https://eliminateadultacne.com/resources

Metabolic Type® and Metabolic Typing® are Registered Trademarks of Healthexcel, Inc. and are used with permission.

If you aren't able to or do not wish to take the Metabolic Typing® Test online, I have listed six different Diet Plans in Appendices 1-6 and ensured I exclude any foods known to cause acne from the lists. Without testing, the only way to find out which foods are causing your acne would be to try each one in turn.

> I have also included all six diet plans at
> https://eliminateadultacne.com/resources

> If you want more detail, I advise you to take the online Metabolic Typing® Test to find out your exact type.

There are also options for simpler tests in William Wolcott's book, *The Metabolic Typing Diet®* or The Primal Pattern Diet Type® questionnaire in Paul Chek's book, *How to Eat, Move & Be Healthy!*

The tests in these books will not give you the level of detail in terms of test results, nor will they give you the same level of advice as the online test.

(Note: I have no financial interest in any of the suggested tests. However, when working with my clients, I do pass on the cost of the online Metabolic Typing® Test to my clients).

Explanation of the diet plans:
If you complete the online test, it will tell you your dominant Metabolic Type®. Some people are oxidiser dominant while others are autonomic dominant.

Oxidiser Dominant:
There are three types of oxidiser dominance:

1. slow oxidiser
2. fast oxidiser
3. mixed oxidiser

Again, though the theory behind these diets is quite complex, I explain them in simpler terms.

The rate of oxidation in the body, in this instance, refers to the speed at which nutrients are converted into energy. A slow oxidiser turns nutrients into energy slowly; a fast oxidiser turns nutrients into energy quickly, and a mixed oxidiser is somewhere in between.

Autonomic Dominant:
There are three types of autonomic dominance:

1. sympathetic

2. parasympathetic

3. balanced.

In simple terms, some people are sympathetic dominant and require foods that push their systems more toward the parasympathetic. Others are parasympathetic dominant and require foods that push their systems toward the sympathetic to maintain balance. A balanced type requires food from both sides to remain in balance.

> For a deeper explanation of Metabolic Typing®, you may wish to read, *The Metabolic Typing Diet* by William Wolcott and Trish Fahey.[218]

Why is this important to understand?

To create optimal energy on the cellular level, which includes the detoxification of cells, a slow oxidiser needs food that is quite easy or fast to digest, whilst a fast oxidiser needs food that takes longer to break down and digest.

In the six Metabolic Typing® diet plans, 'green' foods are 'ideal' foods and should make up most of your diet. 'Black' foods can be eaten in small amounts, while 'red' foods (those with a strikethrough) should be completely avoided.

In the Mixed Oxidiser Diet Plan and the Balanced Type Diet Plan, there are also 'purple' foods. If your type is a mixed oxidiser, you should eat 'purple' foods together and 'green' foods together and try not to mix them in the same meal. This will help maintain optimal blood sugar levels and avoid blood sugar surges that can lead to breakouts.

Metabolic Type® and Metabolic Typing® are Registered Trademarks of Healthexcel, Inc. and are used with permission.

---

[218] 2002

Four-Day Diet Plan

Once you have your list of 'ideal' foods, you can prepare a Four-Day Diet Plan (Appendix 7). Not only will this help you plan what you will eat each day, but it will also provide you with your first grocery-shopping list.

Whilst the template below provides space for five eating opportunities each day, it doesn't mean you have to eat that often. Most people, especially when they are eating right for their 'type', only need to eat between two and four times per day.

When completing your Four-Day Diet Plan, ensure you include all ingredients, such as herbs and spices and fats and oils you may use when cooking meals. Also, try to include some cooked and some raw food.

You will probably need to prepare a Four-Day Diet Plan at the start of each season (spring, summer, autumn/fall and winter), not only because different food will be in season at different times, but also because your desires will change with the seasons, and your Metabolic Type® will also change.

Example diet plans (for each Metabolic Type®) can be found in Appendices 7-12.

Having different diet plans throughout the year will also help prevent boredom and increase the variety of nutrients you consume.

> You can find an electronic version of the Four Day Diet template at https://eliminateadultacne.com/resources

> You can also find examples of completed diet plans for each Metabolic Type® you can use for inspiration at https://eliminateadultacne.com/resources

Fine-tuning

Once you know which foods are right for you, you will need to fine-tune the fats, proteins, and carbohydrates (or macronutrient ratios (MNRs)).

The food we eat affects three main things:

- satiety (feelings of fullness),
- energy levels and
- emotions.

Ideally, one to two hours after eating, we experience a continued feeling of satiety, increased energy levels, and an improvement in our emotional wellbeing.

So, one to two hours after eating, we need to 'check in' to decide whether we are still satiated, have good energy levels and are emotionally uplifted. If not, we are receiving feedback from our body-mind that there was something not quite right in the meal. If you had one or more negative reactions to the meal, such as craving sweets, it might be that you ate too much, didn't eat enough, or had too many carbs or not enough fat, for example.

If you eat a meal, and one to two hours after, you feel great, recognise the makeup of the meal, the size and the proportion of MNRs. The next time you have a meal, try one that is the same size with the same MNRs and see if you experience the same reaction. If you did great, you are finding out what works for you and 'dialling in' to your optimal MNR.

If, however, you experience a negative reaction—such as sweet cravings, hunger, energy crashes, and so on—that's okay. It means you are learning what is not right for you. Perhaps, the next time you have the same meal, try fewer carbohydrates and more fat and protein and note how you respond. If you respond better, great! Perhaps try a bit fewer carbohydrates and more fat and protein the next time and see how you respond. Keep going in that direction until you feel as if you have achieved a less favourable response. When you do, your previous meal was in your 'sweet spot'!

Carbohydrates: found in fruit, vegetables, legumes, (grains), (Dairy)

Proteins: found in meat, poultry, fish, offal, eggs, (dairy)

Fats: found in all the 'protein' foods above plus avocado, extra virgin olive oil, coconut oil, avocado oil, tallow, duck fat, goose fat, butter, ghee, nuts and seeds.

Remember that we are all different, and all of us require different MNRs. You may also discover that you require different MNRs at different times of the day. For instance, you might do great with an almost entirely meat-based breakfast, a more even lunch and a dinner with more carbohydrates than fats and proteins. The only way to find out is by doing!

You can also assess your meals by checking your blood sugar levels with a glucometer (as mentioned previously). The ideal times to check your blood sugar are:

- upon awakening,
- before lunch,
- before dinner and/or
- before bed.

There are two types of glucometers:

- one type is calibrated for blood plasma:
- blood sugar should be between 5.0-5.5 mml/L or 90-100mg/DL
- the other is calibrated for whole blood:
- blood sugar should be between 4.4-5.0 mml/L or 80-90mg/DL

The instruction manual should state which type of glucometer you have.

If the readings are outside of these parameters, it suggests your blood sugar levels are out of balance. Ensuring you eat right for your type is crucial, as is avoiding too much stress (more on that later).

A copy of the Diet Check Record sheet I use with my clients to help them 'fine tune' their diet is available at https://eliminateadultacne.com/resources. These should be used daily until you have totally dialled into your Metabolic Type®.

Metabolic Type® and Metabolic Typing® are Registered Trade-marks of Healthexcel, Inc. and are used with permission.

Food Quality

This section explains why eating high-quality food is essential if you want to give yourself every chance to achieve clear skin. In addition to eating right for your Metabolic Type®, avoiding foods you are sensitive to and eliminating foods known to cause acne, you also need to consider food quality.

Not all food is created equal.

The longest study ever performed on organic versus non-organic produce (a 21-year study by Lady Eve Balfour) has shown that organic soil contains 85% more microorganisms than non-organic soil. It is the microorganisms in the soil that make the nutrients that feed the plants. If there are 85% fewer microorganisms in conventional (non-organic) soils, then it doesn't take a brain surgeon to work out that there'll be considerably fewer nutrients in crops grown in these soils.

What does that have to do with acne?

As I have stated before, it is essential to optimise the level of nutrients available for all your organs and skin to maintain a clear complexion. It is also imperative to minimise toxins in the body as a backup of toxins may end up causing acne. Not only does non-organic produce have a much lower level of nutrients, but it also has dangerous and toxic chemicals such as pesticides, herbicides, fungicides, rodenticides and chemical NPK fertiliser. Many pesticides now contain chemical hormones to prevent pests from reproducing, and as you may be aware, an imbalanced hormonal system can also cause acne (as well as many other disease states).

Eating food containing chemical toxins puts stress on your nervous and hormonal systems in general, further increasing your likelihood of acne.

How to Eat Good Quality

With regards to vegetables (and fruit), eat as much organic produce as possible, ideally 100%. Look for organic certification, such as the Soil Association (in the UK) or speak to your local farmer to ensure they don't use commercial fertilisers, hormones and/or medical drugs or feed their animals unnatural feed.

With regards to meat, look for free-range organic (or even better bio-dynamic), and animals that are fed their natural feed. For instance, many animals are fed grains when it isn't their natural diet. Chickens, for instance, naturally live off grass, worms and insects, whilst cows and sheep naturally eat grass, not wheat, corn or soy, which is cheap and used to fatten them up quickly and easily. The problem with unnatural diets is that it makes the animals toxic and sick, and you do not want to eat sick, toxic animals.

With regards to fish, only buy wild fish, not farmed. Farmed fish are fed unnatural feed, swim in their own faeces in confined conditions and are sick. Even if the fish is organic (which means it's fed organic feed), it is not a healthy fish and will lack nutrients such as omega-3 oils.

Most fish are highly contaminated with mercury and other heavy metals. As larger fish eat smaller fish, it is not advisable to eat large fish, such as tuna or shark.

If you are going to eat fish, choose smaller fish that contain less mercury. If buying salmon, only ever choose Wild Alaskan as the water is cleaner there, and the fish eat a natural diet (unless they are farmed).

A golden rule for eating good quality is to read labels and ask questions of your grocer, butcher, fishmonger or waiter.

Also, as Paul Chek says, "If it wasn't available 10,000 years ago, don't eat it!" Acne didn't exist 10,000 years ago, so don't eat the things that help cause it now.

Preparing to Eat

Apart from eating the right food, you must also be aware of 'how' to eat, too. You might think you know how to eat correctly, but sadly, the truth is that most people do not know how to get the most out of their meals.

In order to fully digest and assimilate our food's nutrients, we need to be in a state of relaxation, also known as a parasympathetic state. We need to ensure we are properly hydrated, which is necessary for our digestive juices to do their jobs.

Apart from what you are about to eat, you must also consider where you are going to eat. Many people eat whilst watching TV or their smart devices or at their desks at work or at home whilst at the computer. None of these places is ideal. Making an effort to sit at a dining table or picnic table (outdoors in nature when the weather allows) is a great start.

Eating whilst doing something that stimulates the mind means you are not switching off and getting into a relaxed state; therefore, you will not be in an optimal state to fully digest your food. You need to ensure your eating environment is relaxed, quiet and as low-stress as you can possibly make it. Relaxing music also helps. Classical music, for instance, has been shown to aid in digestion.

Once you have decided where you are going to eat, drink a glass of high-quality water 15 minutes before starting your meal to hydrate your digestive organs.

Also, prior to the meal, you need to stimulate either the production of hydrochloric acid (HCl) in the stomach or take HCl supplements. Apple cider vinegar and Swedish bitters can be used to help stimulate HCl. I cover more on supplements below.

During the meal, you will also need enzymes (in your small intestines) to adequately break down the food. If you don't have a gallbladder, you'll also need to take some bile salts to help break down the fats in your diet.

Don't worry about the details of these supplements yet—we only look to address them once you are eating correctly.

Another crucial thing is to chew every mouthful of food until it is liquidised before swallowing. The grinding down of food with your teeth breaks it down into its constituent parts while mixing with the enzymes in your saliva to further break down the food to make it easier to digest.

To recap, prior to eating:

- Find a relaxed place to eat away from your normal distractions.
- Drink a glass of good-quality water 15 minutes prior to starting each meal.
- You may need to take HCl, apple cider vinegar, or Swedish bitters prior to the meal.
- You may need to take digestive enzymes (and bile salts if you don't have a gallbladder) during the meal.
- Chew slowly and fully until the food is liquidised before swallowing.

Essential Supplementation

Once you have fine-tuned your macronutrient ratios, the next step is to add in your essential supplements. If you have taken the online Metabolic Typing® Questionnaire, your essential supplements will be stated in your results.

There are four essential supplements required. You might ask, why can't I obtain all the nutrients I need from my diet? That would be a valid question. There are two main reasons we often need dietary supplements:

1. The quality of the food we eat (even organic) is far lower than would have been available 100 years ago.
2. The myriad of stressors we face depletes our nutrient resources.

The following supplements are recommended as essential:

1. digestive enzymes (preferably right for your Metabolic Type®)

2. hydrochloric acid (HCl) (preferably right for your Metabolic Type®)

3. multivitamin and mineral (preferably right for your Metabolic Type®)

4. fish oils (good quality)

Good sources for dietary supplements can be found at
https://eliminateadultacne.com/resources

Digestive enzymes and HCl can, in some cases, require a dose larger than the manufacturer's normal recommendation. Taking the right amount relies on your being aware of how you feel after your meals and adjusting accordingly. More on that later.

HCl is also contraindicated if you have an H Pylori infection, meaning that if you have an H Pylori infection, please do not use HCl acid supplements.

It is standard practise to advise my clients to introduce no more than one supplement at a time. This is to highlight any negative reactions to a particular supplement. Otherwise, if you take more than one new supplement at a time and you have a negative reaction, you simply won't know which one it is. I always advise taking a new supplement for three to five days before introducing another to monitor for any negative reactions.

In my experience, negative reactions to high-quality supplements are rare, but they do happen. I once had a client with negative reactions to the herb ashwagandha, but I've also had many other clients with nothing but positive responses to the same herb. So, with food and supplements, it is always a case of test and see because we are all different. We are all individuals, biochemically.

Quality of Supplements

The quality of supplements is also essential. If you can't afford good quality, organic made from real food supplements, it is better to go without. Poor-quality synthetic supplements are made in a lab, and our immune systems do not recognise them as food, which initiates an immune response and causes inflammation (one of the causes of acne). Like many other things in life, cheap supplements are nearly always poor-quality supplements.

Eliminating Sensitive Foods

Back in 2000, I had a food sensitivity test, and the results suggested I should avoid certain foods. It was also recommended I go on an anti-fungal diet, as I had a Candida albicans overgrowth. After two weeks of avoiding my sensitive foods, my skin cleared greatly. The next five to ten years saw a gradual improvement (as I learned more) to the point where I no longer had breakouts. As a side note, my eczema and hay fever also disappeared after avoiding my sensitive foods and eating right for my Metabolic Type®.

Whilst there appears to be little scientific research into acne and food sensitivities, there is empirical evidence of people's acne improving once they have eliminated sensitive foods.

So how does that work?

To explain this, I need to give you a brief overview of what food sensitivities are.

To explain food sensitivities, I must discuss the immune system, which is:

> a system of biological structures and processes within an organism that protects against disease by identifying and killing pathogens and tumor [sic] cells. It detects a wide variety of agents, from viruses to parasitic worms, and needs to distinguish them from the organism's own healthy cells and tissues in order to function properly.[219]

---

[219] 'Immune System,' 2001

In their book, *Your Hidden Food Allergies Are Making You Fat,*[220] Deutsch and Rivera describe the immune system as:

> teams of specialised cells, some of which contain arsenals of powerful chemicals. The cells are like loyal eager troops of foot soldiers, awaiting instructions from their commanding officers, prepared to defend the body from foreign invaders at a moment's notice. They are armed with chemicals such as histamine and other preformed mediators-typically inactive, but always awaiting the signal that will cause their release. Enter an unfriendly bacteria, virus, parasite, or any foreign substance that the immune system believes might be harmful, and immune cells are brought to attention, prepared to release their chemical weapons to fight the invader.[221]

In the case of food sensitivity, the immune system identifies the food as a pathogen or unfriendly invader, and it stimulates an immune response whenever the food is eaten. When there is an immune response in the body, there is always internal damage and inflammation caused by the release of chemicals called mediators (histamine, prostaglandins, cytokines, etc.) from white blood cells. The damage caused by the immune reaction creates debris that needs to be removed.

So, how does this cause acne?

To date, I'm not aware of any research conducted on food sensitivity and acne (perhaps because there is no profit to be made from food elimination diets).

It is, however, possible that the following may be a link between food sensitivity and acne:

- Mediators are toxic, thereby increasing the toxic load on the body.

---

[220] 2002
[221] 1998

- Debris caused by the destruction of the foods is not effectively eliminated, which increases the toxic load.

- Damage caused by the mediators damages the small intestine, increasing the likelihood of microbes escaping into the bloodstream.

- Damage to the intestinal barrier allows undigested foodstuff, microbes and their toxins to enter the bloodstream and end up in the skin, causing an immune response and inflammation.

- Damage to the intestinal barrier decreases the amount of nutrient uptake, thereby reducing the availability of nutrients to the organs and skin.

- Stimulation of the nervous system could cause an over-reaction to the Cutibacterium acnes bacteria, causing redness and swelling.

Whilst we don't know the link between food sensitivity and acne for sure or the exact mechanism, that doesn't mean there isn't a link. Years ago, there were no scientific links between lung cancer and cigarette smoking or asbestos and asbestosis, but we are very aware of these links today.

Just because the link wasn't fully understood didn't mean people didn't suffer.

All Food Sensitivity Tests Are Not Created Equal

There are many food sensitivity tests available on the market. The technology is constantly being updated and improved as the science in immunology continues to uncover new information. I have used a number of tests over the years. I started using the ALCAT Test, switched to an IgG test, an IgG4 test, and then a Mediator Release Test. Most recently, I've used a test that compares IgE, IgG, IgG4 and Complement responses. For up-to-date information, please check out the resources page on my website (see details below).

'Ig' stands for immunoglobulins, also known as antibodies. These are glycoprotein molecules produced by plasma cells (white blood cells). They are a critical part of the immune response, specifically recognising and binding to particular antigens, such as bacteria or viruses (and sometimes unrecognised foods) and aiding in their destruction.

> Information on food sensitivity testing can be found at
> https://eliminateadultacne.com/resources

Many doctors suggest food intolerance or sensitivity tests aren't accurate. This is true for most of them, but most medical doctors aren't up-to-date on the latest research and technology.

Some food sensitivity tests are inaccurate, and some generate a lot of false positives. This means that many foods are shown as problematic even when they're not. This can lead to a large number of foods being unnecessarily avoided. It can also make eating a good, varied diet difficult, if not impossible.

Pulse Testing

Another option—and one that doesn't cost anything—is a Pulse Test.

Here are the instructions for completing Pulse Testing:

1. Record the name of the food item or supplement to be tested below.

2. Sit quietly for five minutes, then measure your resting pulse rate for one full minute and record it in the pre-test pulse rate column below.

3. Place the food item or supplement you are testing on your tongue and close your mouth. You do not need to chew or swallow the sample—just get a good taste.

   Note: Encapsulated supplements need to be removed from the capsule first.

4. Wait at least one minute.

5. Check your pulse rate again for one full minute.

6. Record the result in the post-test pulse rate column below.

If your pulse rate increases or drops by four or more beats per minute, the item being tested has caused a reaction.

7. Rinse your mouth thoroughly with pure, warm water, and wait until your pulse rate has returned to the pre-test rate.

    Note: This can take hours to happen with severe reactions, but it normally only takes about ten minutes.

8. Repeat this test with the next food item or supplement.

Option: Do this test after eating a whole meal. An increase or drop indicates something in the meal is causing a reaction. Note all food items eaten, then test them individually at the next meal or at a later time.

The advantage of using the Pulse Test is that there is no expense. It does, however, take some time. The decision is yours as to whether you arrange a blood test or perform the Pulse Test!

Appendix 14 includes a table for you to chart your Pulse Test results.

Other Foods to Avoid

In this section, I indicate which foods the research shows have a link to acne. These foods need to be avoided if you want to kiss your acne goodbye and live a carefree, confident life.

I used to use a fantastic software package in my practice called Food Pharmacy®. Sadly, the company no longer exists, but fortunately for you, I did manage to save the important diet plans for acne (Appendices 1-6). The Food Pharmacy software included data on a series of health conditions that have been scientifically researched to determine whether food can cause or exacerbate each condition, and if so, which ones. When I had clients with acne, I plugged in as much information about the client as possible (their Metabolic Type®, sensitive foods, etc.), ticked the 'acne vulgaris/rosacea' button, and the software worked out the ideal Diet Plan for the person (see Diet Plan in Appendix 15–note: this isn't for any particular Metabolic Type®).

In the Acne Elimination Diet Plan in Appendix 15, the example foods are shown in 'green', 'black', 'italics' and 'red'.

Green foods do not exacerbate acne. These are the foods you should eat most of the time, as they generally help with acne. Green foods should make up the majority of your diet.

Black foods are neutral where acne is concerned, and they can be eaten, but try to focus mainly on green foods.

Foods in italics might increase the likelihood of acne and should be eaten very sparingly.

Research shows that red foods cause acne, and they should be completely avoided. Acne is linked to the hormone insulin (secreted when blood sugar increases), so foods high in sugar are shown as something to avoid below. Food like some fruit, most grains, starchy vegetables and all sugar-containing foods and drinks should also be avoided.

If you took the online Metabolic Typing® Questionnaire and have received your results, you should have received your diet plan specific to your Metabolic Type®. What you need to do now is cross out any foods listed below, plus any foods similar to those listed below, such as any dairy and sugary foods. You can also refer to the relevant diet plan in the appendices (also available at https://eliminateadultacne.com/resources)

Metabolic Type® and Metabolic Typing® are Registered Trade-marks of Healthexcel, Inc. and used with permission.

Here Is a List of Foods Shown to Exacerbate Acne	
Dairy	Blue Cheese, Brie, Buttermilk, Camembert, Cheddar, Colby, Cottage Cheese, Cream, Edam, Feta, Goat Cheese, Goat Milk, Gouda, Gruyere, Ice Cream, Milk, Monterey Jack, Mozzarella, Muenster, Neufchatel, Parmesan, Provolone, Ricotta, Romano, Roquefort, Sorbet, Sour Cream, Swiss Cheese, Whey, Yogurt
Legumes	Black-eyed Peas
Beverages	Beer, Fruit Juice, Rice Milk, Soft Drinks (colas), Spirits, Wine
Grains	Barley, Buckwheat, Millet, Oats, Rice, Rye, Wheat
Vegetables	Beetroot, Butternut Squash, Potato, Summer Squash, Sweet Potato, Sweet Corn, Tomatoes
Fruit	Bananas, Cantaloupe, Dates, Figs, Pineapple, Raisins, Watermelon
Oils & Fats	Margarine
Herbs, Spices & Seasoning	Chocolate, Honey, Ketchup, Sugar

Referenced from: Food Pharmacy® Software.

In addition, other oils and fats that can cause inflammation/acne and should, therefore, also be avoided are:

- corn oil
- cottonseed oil
- peanut oil
- safflower oil
- sesame oil
- sunflower oil

When you buy fats and oils, ensure they are organic. Buy only cold-pressed oils. Do not buy oils in clear glass as light will destroy it, and plastic bottles leach plastic into the oil.

All fats and oils, including fish oils, should taste and smell 'fresh'. If they do not, dispose of them. Rancid fats and oils are extremely toxic and interfere with normal fatty acid metabolism severely.

When doing grocery shopping, it is so important to check labels to ensure the ingredients do not include acne-causing foods. When eating out, ask the waiter to ensure that none of these offending foods are in your meal. Most restaurants today are very good at using alternative ingredients.

Wherever possible, use single-ingredient foods to make meals, such as apples, beef, broccoli, avocado and so on. There are no labels to check with these food items, but if you are buying in a store, it is worth checking whether they have added ingredients. I was once shocked when buying beef in a well-known 'health food' store in the USA that sugar was an added ingredient. Luckily, I checked the label and put it back on the shelf.

Some healthy oils you can use and cook with include:

- coconut oil
- beef tallow
- duck fat
- goose fat
- avocado oil
- lard
- butter and ghee (some people can have this without causing acne)

Once you have your diet plan and a list of food, you can do your grocery shopping. At the beginning of the process, it is crucial to stick to the plan, being vigilant to avoid disappointment.

This is also a good time to look back at the section entitled Plan to Overcome Obstacles Before They Arise to ensure that once you start the process, you will maximise your chance of success by planning to avoid unnecessary pitfalls and setbacks.

Hydration Recommendations

How much water should you drink each day?

Your daily intake of water depends on your weight. To calculate the amount you require, you have two options. Take your body weight in pounds or kilograms and use the table below to calculate your minimum daily water intake.

Daily Drinking Water Amounts			
Imperial		Metric	
Bodyweight (lbs.)	Water Intake (ounces)	Bodyweight (kgs)	Water Intake (litres)
120	60	55	1.8
125	62.5	57.5	1.9
130	65	60	2.0
135	67.5	62.5	2.1
140	70	65	2.1
145	72.5	67.5	2.2
150	75	70	2.3
155	77.5	72.5	2.4
160	80	75	2.5
165	82.5	77.5	2.6
170	85	80	2.6
175	87.5	82.5	2.7

180	90	85	2.8
185	92.5	87.5	2.9
190	95	90	3.0
195	97.5	92.5	3.1
200	100	95	3.1
205	102.5	97.5	3.2
210	105	100	3.3
215	107.5	102.5	3.4
220	110	105	3.5
225	112.5	107.5	3.5
230	115	110	3.6

These are the minimal amounts. If you exercise, are in a warm climate, drink alcohol, smoke cigarettes or drink caffeinated drinks, you may need more than the suggested amounts.

Water Quality

It's not just about the amount of water; it's also about getting the right quality of water. If you think drinking tap water will get the job done, think again.

Almost everywhere today, chemicals are added to tap water to make it 'safer' to drink. However, tap water has been found to include chlorine, fluoride, pesticide residues and traces of female contraceptives, to name just a few.

Chlorine is added to the water in the form of sodium hypochlorite, also known as household bleach. Sodium hypochlorite is added to the water to kill any bugs in the water supply. It is, however, highly toxic and despite what experts might say about the safety of low levels of chlorine in our water supply, it can be dangerous.

Chlorine also kills the good bacteria in your gut. This means that bad bacteria, fungi and parasites are free to roam, taking over your gut. These bugs prevent you from absorbing all the nutrients in your food and poison your gut. There are also chlorine-resistant bugs, like Giardia Lamblia, which is a known chlorine-resistant parasite. This means that chlorine can't completely eliminate all the bugs anyway, and for that reason alone, it is not worth using tap water.

Fluoride is added to some municipal water supplies as it allegedly helps with bone and tooth health. However, it has been suggested that fluoride does more damage to bone than it helps. Fluoride, like chlorine, is highly toxic, and its safety has been brought into serious question by many experts, particularly by Christopher Bryson in his book *The Fluoride Deception*.[222] Again, another good reason not to use tap water!

We also know that hormones play a role in acne, so drinking and washing in water containing traces of synthetic female hormones from contraceptives only serves to further destabilise your hormonal system, making it harder to get your skin under control.

The residues of chemical fertilisers found in tap water today is not only toxic, but it also interrupts your hormonal system's balance and puts your detoxification pathways under more stress.

So, what's the alternative?

I suggest to my clients that the best water to drink is reverse osmosis (RO) filtered, but there is a caveat to that: once the water has been filtered, it MUST be remineralised before use as the filtering process is so thorough it eliminates most minerals from the water, and without minerals, the water is extremely acidic.

Drinking pure water can draw minerals from your bones and teeth, increasing your chance of osteoporosis and dental problems.

You can buy RO systems for your house for a few hundred dollars. At the time I had my system fitted at home, I was spending around

---

[222] 2006

£500 ($625) per year on bottled water. Not only did I save a lot of money, but I also stopped using a lot of plastic bottles each year, which are not good for your skin or the environment.

If you use RO-filtered water, there are a few options for remineralising the water:

- Add a little organic, unprocessed sea salt to the water.
- Add liquid minerals to the water (I use Perfect Minerals).
- Use a filter that remineralises the water.

I use the Aqua Tru home system and prefer a remineralising filter, as I find it tastes better, lasts longer, and is more convenient than adding liquid minerals.

If you add sea salt to the filtered water and can taste the salt in the water, you have added too much. For most, one pinch of salt for each litre of water (34 ounces) is normally about enough. Normal table salt will not do the trick. Table salt only contains sodium and chloride and will not give you the minerals your body needs.

If you are unable to drink RO-filtered water, the next best thing is good quality spring water. Evian and Vittel are possibly the best brands based on their mineral content. You should generally go for a minimum of 300 mg/L of dry mineral residue. This is shown on the label of the product.

Where possible, buy mineral water in glass bottles to avoid contamination from the plastic bottle, not to mention damaging the environment.

Other brands that are not as high in mineral content but of reasonable quality are Fiji, Buxton and Highland Spring. You can add a little organic, unprocessed sea salt or liquid minerals to these to bring them up to adequate mineral levels.

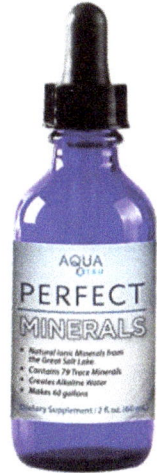

Dehydration Reduction Plan

In addition to increasing hydration levels, you must reduce dehydrating beverages.

Many beverages today take more water out of the system than they put in. Some are diuretics (increasing the rate of the elimination of water), whilst others are so high in sugar they take more water to process in the digestive system than they add to the body.

Common diuretic beverages include caffeinated drinks, such as coffee, tea, cola, energy drinks and all alcoholic beverages. In addition to being diuretics, caffeinated drinks stimulate your stress hormones and can upset your hormone balance over time. If a hormonal imbalance is causing your acne, then caffeinated drinks will not help you. In addition, coffee beans are one of the most highly-sprayed crops with pesticides. This means your coffee beans are toxic. If you drink coffee, I highly recommend you only ever drink certified organic. Many sports and energy drinks contain caffeine. These drinks also contain sugar or artificial sweeteners. Candace Pert, PhD, author of *Molecules of Emotion*,[223] states that sugar, 'Is more unhealthy and more addictive than heroin.' Also, sports drinks quickly raise insulin levels. We know there is a direct link between insulin and acne, so for this reason, it is worth not using sports drinks unless you're a professional athlete.

Artificial sweeteners, on the other hand, have been shown to be toxic and disrupt or kill brain and nerve cells. The movie *Sweet Misery: A Poisoned World* by Cori Brackett and JT Waldron shows several people whose lives have been ruined through the use of artificial sweeteners, many of which have severe neurological disorders.

When it comes to caffeinated drinks, it is not recommended to stop immediately. Caffeine is a powerful drug, and the withdrawal symptoms can be unpleasant. I suggest my clients slowly reduce caffeine intake over a series of weeks. I always suggest they begin by eliminating the caffeinated drink taken the latest in the day first, then the next latest and so on.

---

[223] 1999

A coffee reduction schedule might look like this:

Week	8am	10am	1pm	3pm	7pm	10pm
1	√	√	√	√	√	√
2	√	√	√	√	√	
3	√	√	√	√		
4	√	√	√			
5	√	√				
6	√					

√ - denotes a cup of coffee

As you can see, as the weeks go by, the latest caffeinated drink of the day is dropped until only the first one of the day is drunk. Ideally, no caffeine should be consumed, but for some die-hard caffeine drinkers, one coffee or tea first thing in the morning isn't so bad. It ties in with the time of the day your stress hormones are highest, so it is much better than drinking in the evening when your adrenal glands (which secrete stress hormones) are trying to rest.

As I said before, if you are going to drink coffee, it must be certified organic.

For the best results and to follow this plan correctly and effectively, only good quality water and some herbal teas should be drunk.

You might wish to use a similar schedule to wean yourself off sodas, fizzy drinks or fruit juices. Just replace each of those drinks with good-quality water or herbal tea.

With regards to alcohol, my suggestion is to stop completely for 12 weeks if you are serious about getting results. Alcohol is a poison and a diuretic. Alcohol also plays havoc with blood sugar levels, and we know fluctuating blood sugar and insulin levels are linked to acne.

If you're reading this and thinking, 'Oh, my, that's going to be impossible,' then I have these words of advice for you. If peer pressure or social or work situations are making it hard to avoid alcohol, you need to take a reality check. In reality, you need to take responsibility for yourself and learn to be happy with who you are, not worry about what others think of you and remember how important it is for you to get clear skin.

If you drink alcohol every day, then you might need to understand what unmet needs you have that the alcohol is helping you avoid. If you feel that giving up alcohol is going to be challenging, then I suggest seeking professional help.

Chapter summary/Key takeaways

In summary:

- Metabolic Typing® is the process of identifying and fine-tuning a diet that is right for you, not just for your skin, but for your whole-body health.

- Metabolic Typing® includes eating the right proportion of fats, proteins and carbohydrates for your individual needs to optimise cellular energy and cellular detoxification.

- You can discover your Metabolic Type® by taking the online test, or if you prefer, you can take a more basic test in William Wolcott's book *The Metabolic Typing Diet* or the Primal Pattern® Diet Typing questionnaire in Paul Chek's book *How to Eat, Move & Be Healthy!*[224]

- In addition to eating right for your 'type', you must also ensure to eliminate any food you are sensitive to. You can take a blood test to establish the foods you are sensitive to, or you can perform a Pulse Test on all the food you consume.

---

[224] 2004

- In addition to eating right for your 'type' and eliminating food you are sensitive to, you must also eliminate any food known to cause acne.

- You should also consider where you eat your meals to ensure you maximise your ability to digest and assimilate the nutrients.

- Prepare a Four-Day Diet Plan for each season.

- Make sure your food is free-range organic and/or biodynamic.

- Have a plan in place to avoid potential pitfalls or stumbling blocks moving forwards—the plan will only work if you follow it to the T!

- Fine-tune your MNRs by tuning in to how you feel one to two hours after each meal. Use Diet Check Record Sheets to help you with the fine-tuning.

- A minimum amount of clean, mineralised water should be drunk each day depending on your weight, activity levels and the climate. Tap water should be avoided or filtered.

- If required, a water-intake plan should be devised, and daily increases should be no more than an extra half a litre or five ounces daily per week. If required, a plan should be put in place to slowly reduce diuretics, such as caffeine, sports drinks and alcohol.

- If required, introduce a dehydration reduction plan.

In the next chapter, you will learn how about stress, sleep and rest.

SUCCESS STORY 2

Meet Holly.

Holly was a 28-year-old personal trainer suffering from acne when she first came to see me. Holly had terrible breakouts and felt embarrassed and like a 'fraud' when training her clients, as she didn't think she was the perfect example of what it meant to be healthy. Even though she was a personal trainer and trained in nutrition, she didn't realise the food she ate caused her acne and affected her overall health.

Following a few lab tests, it was discovered that Holly had fungal and parasite infections as well as food sensitivities to gliadin (gluten), egg and soy.

Holly changed her diet as advised, following her Metabolic Typing® diet, eliminating sensitive foods and following a plan to reduce her fungal and parasite infections to help heal her gut.

The programme worked a treat for Holly, and she was completely spot-free relatively quickly once the programme was in full flow. She now has much more confidence, especially at work, enjoys her social life and no longer has to wear makeup to go out of the house, which she really loves.

STRESS, SLEEP AND REST

'Tired minds don't plan well. Sleep first, plan later.'

Walter Reisch

Stress

In Part I of this book, I explained how stress can contribute to 'leaky gut syndrome', which allows intestinal contents, including pathogens and toxins, to enter the bloodstream and travel to the skin for excretion. Many believe these pathogens and toxins cause acne whilst excreted through the skin.

When we are stressed, we release stress hormones, especially cortisol, which is released from the adrenal glands. One of cortisol's functions is to break down muscle tissue to release glycogen (sugar stored in the muscle), increasing blood sugar for 'fight or flight'. However, if we are not in a situation where we need to fight or run, the blood sugar doesn't get used. Insulin is then secreted by the pancreas to reduce blood sugar levels, and we know from Part I of this book that insulin, along with IGF-1, increases the likelihood of acne. It is, therefore, imperative that we minimise all stress in our lives to help balance blood sugar levels and avoid unnecessary spikes, causing a large release of insulin.

Cell Energetics

Bone Turnover

Memory and Learning

Glucose Homeostasis — CHO Metabolism

Muscle Integrity — Musculo-skeletal Health — Connective Tissue Turnover

Neural Tissue Health — Neuronal Connectivity

Pro/Anti Inflammatory State

Adrenal Glands

Cortisol to DHEA Ratio

Adrenal Glands

Quality of Sleep and Mood

Eicosanoid Modulation

Immune Regulation

Pancreas - Insulin

Heavy Metal Endo Chelation — Detox. Capacity

Protein Turnover — Fat and Protein Metabolism — Mucosal Surface Integrity (1st-line Immune Defense)

Endocrine Function — Thyroid Function

Mixed Function Oxidase Modulation

Weight and Fat Distribution

Ovarian Hormone Levels

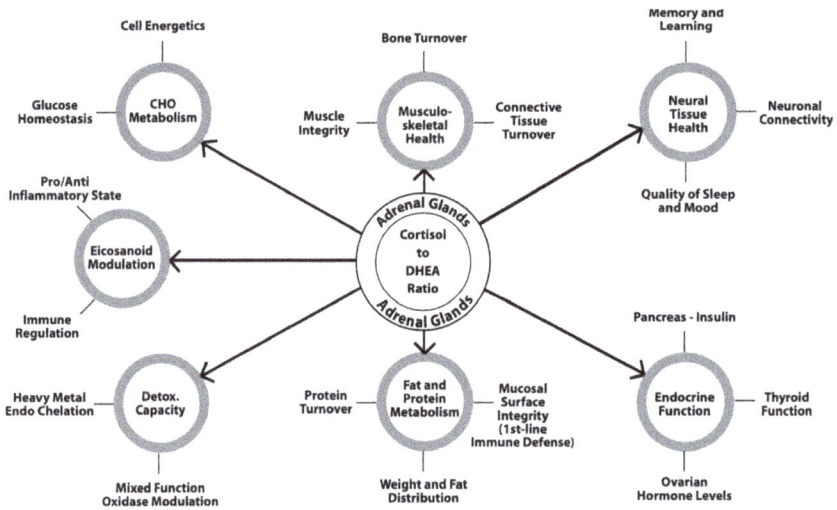

The above illustration[225] shows the physiological connection between the ratio of cortisol to the hormone dehydroepiandrosterone (DHEA), a precursor hormone to the male and female steroid hormones testosterone and oestrogen. When stressed, cortisol levels go up, and DHEA levels tend to lower. Stress causes an imbalance in the optimal ratio between cortisol and DHEA.

What does this have to do with acne?

If you look at the illustration above, when the ratio between cortisol and DHEA is suboptimal, it can affect many other physiological systems. Systems directly affecting acne are glucose homeostasis, quality of sleep, pancreas function, ovarian hormone levels (in females), protein turnover, detoxification capacity (including heavy metal chelation) and immune regulation.

In addition, when we are in a stressed state, blood flow is shunted from the internal organs to our muscles to enable fight or flight. This diversion of blood flowing away from the organs reduces digestion and detoxification and can cause constipation. The reduced ability to digest

---

225 'Biomatrix,' 2000

your food also reduces nutrient availability to your organs—including your skin—and reduces detoxification and an increase of toxic waste in the body, further increasing the likelihood of breakouts. The colon works by squeezing your stools to release water from the stool to help maintain hydration levels. However, if the stool isn't moving through as it should, the squeezing releases toxins into the bloodstream. This is known as autointoxication, which further increases toxicity levels in the body and the likelihood of a breakout.

It should be clear that stress is not helpful to your skin. It is also important to be aware of all the stress you are exposed to. It isn't just mental stress, but any kind of stress that needs to be minimised.

In the book, *How to Eat, Move & Be Healthy*,[226] Paul Chek suggests there are six main types of stress:

1. Physical
2. Chemical
3. Electromagnetic
4. Psychic/Emotional
5. Nutritional
6. Thermal

Whilst it is essential to have some level of stress in each of these areas, it is important to minimise or avoid excessive stress in each and all of them.

Physical stress in the form of exercise is crucial to keep your bones, muscles, heart and lungs in good shape. A lack of exercise causes these tissues and organs to weaken, putting our health at risk. However, too much exercise or exercising with poor posture causes too much stress on the system, especially without enough rest.

---

[226] 2004

Chemical stress is important for our bodies to maintain optimal hormone levels, protein synthesis and energy production. However, in today's world, we are bombarded with thousands of unnatural toxic chemicals our bodies simply did not evolve to deal with. These toxic chemicals need to be avoided wherever possible and safely excreted from the body, which is covered in Chapters 7 and 8.

Electromagnetic stress is essential for life. The sun provides electromagnetic waves essential to all life on Earth. However, we can get too much or not enough sun. Too much can cause our skin to burn, and not enough can cause depression and vitamin D deficiencies. We also have a myriad of modern technology the human body did not evolve to deal with that cause a huge amount of stress to the body. Devices such as mobile phones and towers, tablets, laptops, smart TVs, smart meters, smart watches, electric toothbrushes, hair dryers, Wi-Fi, microwave ovens and poorly fitted or maintained electricity cabling are a few of these devices.

Psychic or mental stress is crucial for our brain development, learning, and enjoyment in life. However, toxic relationships, financial worries and work stress can all cause stress responses in the body. Chapter 3 covered some techniques that can be used to reduce mental stress. Techniques such as meditation, journaling, art therapy, sound therapy, massage, aromatherapy, yoga, tai chi and qi gong can all help to reduce mental stress when performed regularly and frequently.

Nutritional stress is crucial for digesting, assimilating and metabolising nutrients from food. However, over- or under-eating, eating incorrectly for your Metabolic Type® or eating food that has been grown or raised using chemical fertilisers, pesticides, antibiotics, preservatives or colourings causes excess stress. Eating correctly was covered in detail in Chapter 4.

Thermal stress is crucial for helping with your ability to maintain an optimal body temperature of 37°C. The use of cold and heat therapy has become popular in recent years, especially cold plunges or showers and saunas. Giving the body a little heat stress enables it to regulate temperature in times of extreme weather, plus a whole myriad of health benefits. Just like a little exercise stresses the tissues to make them more robust, cold and heat therapies make the body more robust and able to handle stress. However, being in extreme heat, cold or sunlight for too long also causes excessive stress and should be avoided.

When working with clients, I sometimes run a 24-hour Cortisol Rhythm Test, which identifies the amount of cortisol (stress hormone) output at different times of the day. This gives insight into the level of stress the person is under. Whilst not essential, they can be useful in most cases to see how the adrenal glands cope with a person's lifestyle. Re-testing can be useful for charting progress.

However, the most important aspect is to minimise stress using the suggestions in this chapter and the rest of Part II of this book.

It is crucial to identify all stressors in your life and environment and do all you can to remove or reduce them. In the case of chemical toxins, it is also important to safely eliminate them from the body; this is covered in Chapter 7 and Chapter 8.

Sleep and Rest

For millions of years, humans evolved in alignment with sunrise and sundown. Our natural daily hormonal rhythms and nervous system activation are intimately tied to our exposure to sunlight. This is important to understand, not just because acne can be caused by hormones, but because of an even more important reason. As I mentioned in Part I of the book, acne is a sign of an imbalance of bodily systems. When we live our lives differently from how we evolved, it causes stress on the body, and when the stress reaches a certain limit, we experience symptoms, and acne is one of them.

It is important to give our bodies every opportunity to heal as best they can. However, when we apply excessive stress to our bodies, they are not in a position to heal.

The diagram below is taken from the book *How to Eat, Move & Be Healthy!*[227] by Paul Chek. It illustrates these key points:

- At sunrise, when the sun stimulates light receptors in our skin and eyes, stress hormone (shown by the black line) levels increase, especially cortisol. This helps wake us up, get us going for the day, and in years gone by, would have helped us hunt for food.

- After 8.30 am, these stress hormones naturally decline and by sundown, are at their lowest levels.

- After dark, these stress hormone levels stay low, allowing us to rest, repair and recover from the day, both physically (between 10 pm-2 am) and mentally (between 2 am-6 am).

- Conversely, our growth and repair hormones (shown by the white line) remain low during the day whilst we are active but increase after sundown as long as we are in a dark environment and resting. This is how humans lived for millions of years prior to industrialisation.

With our modern lifestyles, nearly all of us tend to have exaggerated stress levels working long hours, having stressful jobs we don't enjoy, relationship and family/parenting challenges, over- or under-exercising, having poor diets, using artificial lights, mobile communication devices and televisions after dark, and not getting enough good quality sleep.

As you can see in the diagram above, when we experience exaggerated stress responses, we spend far too much of the day where our stress hormones are elevated, and our growth and repair hormones do not have the opportunity to increase. This is because the body thinks it is in a state of stress, also known as fight or flight.

When in a state of stress, whether it is truly a matter of life and death or due to an argument with your spouse, the fear of losing your job, or staying up late watching television or flicking through social media, the response is the same.

---

[227] Reproduced with permission (2004).

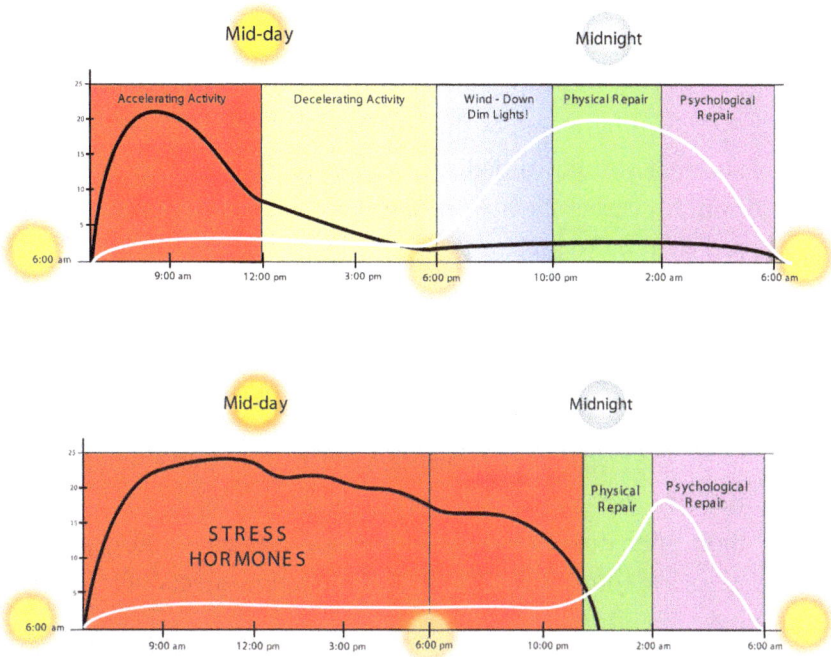

Remember that when in a stressed state, our bodies break down muscle tissue to release muscle glycogen (sugar), which increases the amount of blood sugar to help you run or fight. It also upsets the cortisol-to-DHEA ratio, which then disturbs a number of physiological functions directly related to acne. As an acne sufferer, as mentioned in Part I, you should avoid spiking your blood sugar.

In addition, not resting and getting an adequate amount of sleep throws your hormones out of balance, and as I'm sure you're aware, as an acne sufferer, you want to keep your hormone levels ideal. Another important aspect of too much stress and a lack of sleep is that you physically recover between 10 pm and 2 am, when you are asleep in a dark environment. Physical recovery includes the recovery of your organs, including your skin, other organs of detoxification and your gut; you will soon discover the importance of this.

Sleep Advice

In order to get an optimal night's sleep, here are my recommendations:

- Be in bed by 10 pm at the latest and asleep by 10.30 pm at the latest. If you go to bed much later than 10 pm, go to bed 15 minutes earlier each week until you are able to go to bed and feel tired by 10 pm.

- Avoid ALL unnatural light at least one hour before bed. If you use any unnatural light after dusk, your body thinks it is day-time and will continue releasing stress hormones. This will prevent you from winding down, and your growth and repair hormones will not be at an adequate level to make repairs from the day. Beeswax candles are a great alternative to unnatural light after dusk. Blue light-blocking glasses are also good at negating some but not all of the negative effects of unnatural light after dusk.

- Do not have any electronic devices anywhere in your bed-room as they affect your sleep, even if not switched on. This includes any kind of standby lights (often found on TVs) and electronic alarm clocks. Turn off all electrical sockets in your bedroom—even better, remove the fuse supplying electricity to your bedroom at night.

- Your bedroom must be completely pitch dark at night. Black-out curtains can help to make your room completely dark.

- Have a pre-bed routine to help you unwind for the day. My clients report activities such as having a relaxing bath, listening to relaxing music, having a massage, a sauna, stretching, read-ing, listening to a podcast in the dark, and even taking a cold shower.

- Mobile electronic devices that track your quality of sleep are not recommended.

- Your wifi should be switched off at night.

- Sleeping on a grounding or earthing mat will also help with sleep as it helps dump free radicals from the body throughout the night.

Chapter summary/Key takeaways

In summary:

- It is crucial to minimise excessive stress on the body to help:
    o maintain balanced blood sugar levels avoiding blood sugar spikes,
    o balance cortisol to DHEA ratios and
    o aid detoxification processes.
- There are six main types of stress:
    o physical
    o chemical
    o electromagnetic
    o psychic or mental
    o nutritional
    o thermal
- Our natural daily hormonal rhythms and nervous system activation are intimately tied in with our exposure to sunlight.
- Our bodies and skin repair at night between 10 pm and 2 am when we are asleep in a fully dark room.
- It is important to get to bed on time and sleep for at least eight hours every night.
- Ensure all electronic devices are turned off and that none are in your bedroom whilst you're asleep.
- Switch off your wifi at night.
- Preferably sleep on a grounding or earthing sheet.

The next chapter explains how to balance the Gut-Skin Axis.

SUCCESS STORY 3:

Meet Sharon.

Sharon was a 52-year-old who worked in finance. She had unpredictable breakouts and suffered from stomach pains, was exhausted, and had insomnia.

Following lab testing, it was found that she had a leaky gut, minor infections, HPA Axis dysregulation (she was chronically stressed) and a range of food sensitivities.

Sharon followed my advice with diet and lifestyle changes, including the elimination of sensitive foods and supplementation to help heal the gut and support adrenal function.

Sharon began to feel so much better within days. She is now sleeping through the night, which she is ecstatic about. Her stomach pain has vanished, her skin is consistently great, her energy levels increased, and her weight, particularly around her middle, reduced with what she described as 'absolutely no effort on my part, other than following Leigh's revised eating regime.'

This is a great example of how some people's situations are relatively easily and quickly resolved.

BALANCING THE GUT-SKIN AXIS

'The surface of a human being, then, is not just their skin,
but the twists and turns, furrows and folds
of their inner tube as well.

No matter if it's inner or outer, all of this surface is
potential real estate for microbes.'

Allana Collen

In Chapter 2, I introduced the concept of The Gut-Skin-Axis, explaining the connection and inter-relationship between the gut and your skin. The Gut-Skin-Axis is important for a number of reasons. Firstly, a good intestinal ecology means you can digest and assimilate most, if not all, of the nutrients from your food, supplying your skin with most, if not all, of the nutrients it needs. When I say ecology, I mean the microorganisms residing in the human body. It is believed the human body has 100 trillion cells, 90 trillion of which are microorganisms. Microorganisms residing within us can include viruses, bacteria, fungi and parasites (worms).

Secondly, 'bad' microorganisms can reproduce very quickly, boring holes in your organs (to lay eggs), changing your taste buds, controlling your appetite, eating the food you eat, robbing you of the nutrients, altering your delicate pH balance, creating cellular damage and leaving a lot of toxins behind for your liver to deal with.

Some research shows bacteria other than Cutibacterium Acnes cause acne, such as the Helicobacter Pylori bacteria, believed to infect more than 50% of humans around the world.

As we discussed before, we want to minimise the toxic load on the system to reduce the likelihood of breakouts. In a truly healthy person, there are more beneficial microbes (80%) than unfriendly microbes (20%). When a person has a higher than optimal proportion of unfriendly microbes than beneficial ones, the person is said to have dysbiosis. If you have acne, it is likely you have gut and/or skin dysbiosis.

I often run a stool test to analyse the makeup of my clients' gut microbiome, particularly the GI Map and GI Ecologix. I discuss testing in more detail a little later.

Probiotics for Acne Support

There have been a number of studies illustrating the benefits of probiotic supplementation for reducing levels of IGF-1 and a reduction in acne symptoms. One study suggested Insulin-like Growth Factor-1 (IGF-1) appears to play a role in acne pathogenesis. Therefore, dairy consumption may be associated with the development of acne by promoting IGF-1.[228]

Another study suggests that the addition of Lactobacillus to milk during the fermentation process may help to lower levels of IGF-1, suggesting that probiotics may improve acne by decreasing levels of IGF-1.[229]

A small Italian study investigating the use of *L. acidophilus* and *Bifidobacterium bifidum* noted reduced acne in participants taking the probiotic combination, as well as improved oral tolerance for antibiotics in the same participants.[230]

---

[228] Kober & Bowe, 2015

[229] Marchetti et al., 1987

[230] Scourboutakos et al., 2017

It has also been documented that in addition to a minocycline regimen, probiotic supplementation may further reduce acne lesion count compared to antibiotic use alone.[231] While the evaluation of these acne studies is difficult, they suggest that oral probiotics may play a role as part of combined therapy. It also suggests that acne sufferers achieve better results when taking specific types of probiotics, particularly *L. acidophilus* and *Bifdiobacterium bifidum*. To me, it also suggests that most, if not all, acne sufferers have an imbalanced gut microbiome. Therefore, taking a probiotic containing *L. acidophilus* and *Bifidobacterium bifidum* (if you have acne) would be a sensible move.

Food that Supports the Gut Microbiome

Probiotic food, including fermented food containing live active microbes, such as yoghurt, kefir, miso, kimchi, and sauerkraut.[232] Prebiotics are non-digestible components of food, such as fibre, that can influence the activity of gut microbes thereby mediating host health,[233] such as inulin, arabinogalactan, and guar gum.[234, 235] Be careful if you use yoghurt or kefir as they are dairy products and may cause breakouts in some people. You might be okay with these fermented versions of dairy products, but the only way to know is to try and see once you have your skin under control.

Anti-inflammatory Short Chain Fatty Acids (SCFAs) are produced via the fermentation of prebiotics by commensal (friendly) gut microbes. SCFAs lower the production of the toxic products of fermentation, improve the Th1/Th2 ratio, and increase secretion of IgA in the gut.[236] Therefore, prebiotic foods help reduce toxin levels, optimise the immune system and reduce the likelihood of acne.

---

[231] Scourboutakos et al., 2017

[232] Tuohy et al., 2010

[233] 'Larch Arabinogalactan,' n.d.

[234] Mudgil et al., 2018

[235] Rusu et al., 2019

[236] Chen et al., 2019, p. 1225

Though there are many prebiotic supplements available, a food-first approach is preferred. Food rich in prebiotics include chicory, Jerusalem artichoke, garlic, onions, shallots and spring onion, leeks, chickpeas, lentils, beans, bananas, grapefruit, almonds, flaxseed, bran, and oats.[237] Of course, you still need to avoid prebiotic food that may cause acne, such as bananas, grapefruit and oats.

Because many prebiotic-rich foods are considered fermentable FODMAP foods, they can contribute to gastrointestinal symptoms and may, therefore, be contraindicated in certain individuals for a period of time.[238]

> *FODMAP stands for Fermentable-Oligosaccharides-Disaccharides-Monosaccharides and Polyols.*

If we improve the gut microbiome, the research tends to suggest, for whatever reason, it has a positive effect on acne. Could it be this it is due to healing a 'leaky gut', or is it due to reducing toxic LPS levels and IGF-1 or a combination of these factors?

We can't say with any certainty at the time of writing this book. What is clear is that optimising the gut microbiome has a positive effect on acne.

Stool Testing

It can be helpful to use stool testing when assessing the health of your gut microbiome. This is something I frequently do with my clients to obtain a good understanding of their status, and more accurately, balance of the microbes in their guts. These tests often also look for things like digestive and immune status, which can be helpful when advising clients on how best to balance their gut microbiomes.

---

[237] Sloan et al., 2018

[238] Sturniolo et al., 2001

Two of the best tests available are the GI Map and GI Ecologix. You normally need to work with a professional to obtain these tests. They will also analyse the results and provide suggestions based on the results and you as an individual. There have been times when, without information gathered from these types of tests, I'm not sure if I would have been able to help some of the clients I have worked with over the years. If, however, you're on a budget, I recommend completing ALL of the action points in this book first, and then, if you still need further improvements, consider doing one of these tests.

I will also cover other solutions for helping to reduce the number of pathogenic microbes you might have later in this chapter.

Nutrients to Aid the Gut

A variety of nutrients can be used to decrease gut inflammation and permeability.

Research suggests the use of zinc,[239] glutamine, collagen peptides, glycyrrhizinated liquorice (DGL), curcumin and omega-3 fatty acids.[240, 241, 242,243, 244, 245, 246, 247, 248]

Supporting Digestion

Digestive factors such as hydrochloric acid (HCl) and bile salts are important for maintaining gut microbial health and reversing dysbiosis. Gastric juice is a first-line defence protecting the host against microbes found in saliva and food. An increase in gastric

---

[239] Michielan & D'Incà, 2015

[240] Pugh et al., 2017

[241] Wang et al., 2015

[242] Chen et al., 2017

[243] Frasca et al., 2012

[244] Asha et al., 2017

[245] Shen et al., 2017

[246] Wang et al., 2017

[247] Mani et al., 2013

[248] Lizasa et al., 2015

pH weakens this defence and can allow microbes to survive in the stomach, promoting dysbiosis.[249] Using a betaine HCl supplement may be beneficial if the levels of gastric juices are low. HCl is con-traindicated if *H. pylori* is suspected or confirmed.[250] Apple cider vinegar or Swedish bitters can also be used as an alternative to HCl supplementation.

Bile acids and gut microbes influence each other. Gut microbes modify bile acid homeostasis, and bile acids play a role in maintain-ing gut barrier integrity, regulating commensal bacteria growth and immune system modulation.[251, 252] If you don't have a gallbladder or there is an oily film around your stools, supplementing with Bile Salts is recommended during meals to help digest and assimilate essential fats from your diet.

Balancing the Microbiome

In this section, I show you how to detox heavy metals from the body and specific microbiome-balancing techniques to optimise the ecology of your intestinal tract. I have learned these techniques over the years in my professional training with several organisations, keeping up with the latest research and my clinical practice.

This section teaches you two procedures to help maintain the opti-mal ecology of your gut and minimise the likelihood of acne.

Like the previous chapter, these procedures will only work if you follow the correct Metabolic Type® diet for you and avoid any high-sugar foods.

Note: These procedures are not intended to treat or eradicate any particular condition, virus, fungus, bacteria or parasite.

---

[249] Huang et al., 2017

[250] Kakiyama et al., 2013

[251] Wang et al., 2019

[252] Klinghardt, 2020

Before I walk you through these cleanses, it is important to complete a heavy metal detox. This is because metals in the body protect pathogenic microbes as if they were wearing armour.[253] Any cleanse performed to encourage pathogenic microbes to leave the body is best performed after removing their armour.

Heavy Metal Detox

When coaching clients, where finances allow, I run a lab test for heavy metals. This enables me to see which heavy metals are at toxic levels in the body and monitor the effectiveness of a heavy metal detox. In some cases, when my clients aren't able to run a lab test, I suggest a heavy metal detox, as this is often required for people who suffer from acne. In some cases, it is the cause of their acne and the key to unlocking the door; as soon as the heavy metals were cleared from the client's body, the acne disappeared.

If you can run a heavy metal test, be aware that some metals are often not tested for such as aluminium. This means that even if you are able to run a test and it comes back negative for heavy metals, you might still need a detox. Most heavy metal tests only look for cadmium, lead, mercury and arsenic.

The following protocol[254] is recommended to be carried out for a minimum of 90 days. If you have high levels of toxicity, you may need to detox for a few months longer.

1. HMD Heavy Metal Detox:

HMD is a gentle detoxifier, safe for the entire family and without side effects.

Dosage: 50 drops 3x a day
Children's dosages by weight.
See the complete Dosage Guidelines at https://www.detoxmetals.com/hmd-dosage-guidelines/

---

[253] Kim et al., 2018b

[254] 'What is HMD,' n.d.

2. HMD Lavage:

This herbal drainage remedy has been specifically formulated to open up your detoxification organs and support your kidneys and liver during detox. It will help your body eliminate metals faster and more efficiently and assist in gently and safely flushing out toxins mobilised by HMD.

Dosage: 25 drops 3x day
Children's dosages by weight.
See the complete Dosage Guidelines at https://www.detoxmetals.com/hmd-dosage-guidelines/

3. Organic Chlorella:

Chlorella is ideal for supporting your body during the detoxification program and guaranteeing optimum health.

Dosage: 2 capsules 2x day
Children's dosages by weight.
See the complete Dosage Guidelines at https://www.detoxmetals.com/hmd-dosage-guidelines/

Fluid Intake:
HMD mainly eliminates toxins via the urinary tract; drinking plenty of fluids will ensure your body can effectively flush out all nasty toxins currently stored in your tissues, organs and bones. To further enhance your detox and cleanse your liver, it is recommended to limit your alcohol intake.

When administering HMD and Lavage, it is essential to hold the dropper vertically when counting out the drops for accurate dosing.

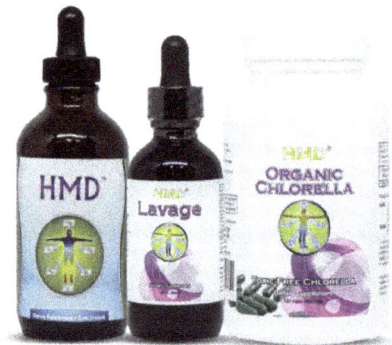

Note: Chlorella is one of a number of binders that act like magnets for toxins. Binders help grab toxins in the intestines and pull them out, aiding in their safe excretion from the body. Binders include.

- Chlorella, which is great for heavy metals of all kinds as well as mycotoxins.
- Zeolite is excellent for mould, mycotoxins and mercury.
- Activated charcoal is broad spectrum (good for all toxins).
- Silica is the most effective binder for removing aluminium from the body.

Binders are great for clearing any type of toxins from the gut, whether it be heavy metals, fungi or parasites.

Due to the overload of toxins in today's environment, it is quite common to recirculate toxins if our livers are overloaded. Binders may be used as an ongoing approach to help in the detoxification process as long as they are of high quality.

Body Ecology Balance

In this section, I show you one of many possible cleanses you can use to optimise your body's ecology.

How Does the Body Ecology Cleanse Work?

The Body Ecology Cleanse works by creating an environment unfavourable to yeast and fungi in the body, colonising your gut with commensal (beneficial) bacteria, and allowing them to proliferate. This reduces the toxic load on the body and skin and allows the uptake and supply of more nutrients to detoxify your skin.

Items that you can use include:

- broad spectrum anti-microbials
- allicin

- oil of oregano
- other antifungal herbs
- probiotics (Lactobacilli and Bifidobacterium or Saccharomyces boulardii)
- prebiotics (PHGG or GOS)

When To Do Them:

- perform the first one after completing a heavy metal cleanse and/or
- once or twice per year

How To Do A Body Ecology Procedure:

The following table lists examples of good-quality brands and products I use in my practice. Other products may be used as long as they are of good quality.

Item	Brand	Product
Biofilm Disruptor	Klaire Labs	Interfase
Broad Spectrum Anti-microbial	Invivo	BioMe Microbia
Anti-microbial – Allicin	Designs for Health	Allicillin
Anti-microbial - Oil of Oregano	Designs for Health	Oil of Oregano
Antifungal Herbs	Raintree Nutrition	Amazon A-F
Probiotic	Invivo	BioMe Barrier or BioMe S. Boulardii
Prebiotics	Invivo	BioMe Pre Bio PHGG and/or BioMe Pre Bio GOS
Polyphenols	Invivo	BioMe Essential

Details of good quality products can be found at
https://eliminateadultacne.com/resources.

Directions:

1. Begin by taking a biofilm disruptor such as Interfase (N-Acetyl-Cystine is also a good biofilm disruptor). Take three to five days before moving on to step two below. Follow the manufacturer's recommendations for dosages.

2. Introduce a broad-spectrum anti-microbial at the lowest dose and build up slowly over a number of days, ensuring you have no negative reactions. Negative reactions are generally rare, but if they do occur, stop using the product for a few days until the symptoms have completely eliminated and re-introduce at the lowest dose. Over time, increase the dose (perhaps every three days) in small increments until you reach the full dose. Smaller people may not require the full dose. Once you have taken the full dose for three days, include step three below. Continue use of the broad-spectrum anti-microbial for four to six weeks.

3. Introduce an anti-microbial or antifungal and follow the same procedure as in step one. Use for six to eight weeks. Once you are taking the full dose, include step four below.

4. Introduce a probiotic (at a different time of day from those above, either first thing in the morning or last thing at night) and follow the same procedure as in step one. Once you are taking the full dose, include step five below. Use the probiotic for at least three to six months and possibly longer.

5. Introduce a prebiotic and follow the same procedure as in step one. These are usually consumed in a hot drink like tea. Start with 1/5 of a teaspoon and increase in increments of 1/5 of a teaspoon. Once you are taking the full dose, continue indefinitely to keep your commensal bacteria fed.

6. Introduce a polyphenol supplement and use it for at least three to six months.

Possible Reactions from the Body Ecology Cleanse

As fungus in the body may 'die off' during this process, you may experience a Herxheimer reaction. This is when more toxins are being released than the detoxification pathways can manage, and toxins build up in the body. When this happens, you might experience toxic or allergy-like reactions, such as bloating, aching, nausea, dizziness, lethargy, headaches, a general feeling of unwellness or a worsening of your acne. This dying-off process usually lasts half a day to a day, but it can last a few days.

Exercise and proper daily bowel movements generally help to reduce the symptoms of the dying-off phase of treatment. Coffee enemas may be helpful for reducing the effects. If you develop dying-off symptoms, don't be concerned, but if they continue, consult your doctor.

Intestinal Cleanse

In this section, I explain a second cleanse you can use to optimise your body ecology.

How Does the Intestinal Cleanse Work?

The Intestinal Cleanse works by creating an environment unfavourable to parasites in the body, thereby reducing your toxic load and enabling you to assimilate more nutrients from your diet, which can only be good for your skin.

What Items Will I Need?

A nutritional supplement product creating an environment unfavourable to parasites. At the time of writing this book, the two products I most frequently recommend are:

- Amazon A-P by Raintree Nutrition or
- Freedom, Cleanse, Restore by PCI

When to do with Them:

- Perform the first cleanse one month after the first Body Ecology Cleanse.
- Perform a subsequent cleanse once a year going forwards.

How to do an Intestinal Cleanse:

1. Begin by taking a Biofilm Disruptor for three to five days before moving on to step two below.
2. Choose one of the two products. If using Amazon A-P, start by taking one capsule once per day and slowly building up to the manufacturer's recommended dose. If using a different product, follow the manufacturer's dosing recommendations.
3. If you experience any unexpected symptoms at any time, halt the cleanse for a day or two until the symptoms have subsided, and build back up slowly.
4. Stay on the cleanse for four to eight weeks or three months for Freedom, Cleanse, Restore once you reach the maximum dose, remembering to pause if you experience symptoms.
5. The use of a daily binder (chlorella, zeolite, and activated charcoal) can also help remove toxins from the body.

Possible Reactions from the Intestinal Cleanse

If parasites are present and dying, you might temporarily experience low energy or flu-like symptoms. If this occurs, come off the program for one or two days to allow your body to detoxify before continuing.

Daily coffee enemas can help eliminate toxins whilst doing the cleanse.

ONCE YOU START AN INTESTINAL CLEANSE, YOU MUST FINISH IT!

THIS IS VERY IMPORTANT!

Details of where you can purchase items required for the Body Ecology Cleanse and Intestinal Cleanse can be found on my website's resources page at https://eliminateadultacne.com/resources

Chapter summary/Key takeaways

In summary:

- There is a lot of research indicating that the use of probiotics helps improve the gut's microbial balance and reduce the severity of acne.

- Foods such as prebiotics and the non-digestible components of food feed the specific bacteria that create short-chain fatty acids aiding in the health of the intestinal wall and helping to prevent a leaky gut.

- Herbal treatments can positively influence the composition of gut microbes.

- Stool Testing can be helpful for assessing gut microbiome. They can help obtain a good understanding of its status, and more accurately, balance of microbes in your gut. These tests often look for things like digestive and immune status, too, which can be helpful for knowing how to best balance your gut microbiome.

- A variety of nutrients can be used to decrease gut inflammation and permeability, such as zinc, glutamine, collagen peptides, deglycyrrhizinated liquorice, curcumin and omega-3 fatty acids.

- Digestion can be supported with the use of HCl, digestive enzymes and bile supplementation. HCl supplementation is contraindicated if you have an H Pylori infection.

- Body Ecology and Intestinal cleanses should be performed once or twice per year.

The next chapter is about the Outside-In Detox.

SUCCESS STORY 4

Meet Litza.

Litza was a 30-year-old professional woman suffering from severe acne and scarring. She was in utter despair and didn't know where to turn. She worried her partner might leave her because of her skin. Litza's condition was as bad as I have ever seen.

Following testing, it was found that Litza had Toxoplasma, as well as food sensitivities to gluten and soy.

Litza was a great client to work with. She jumped in and followed the programme almost 100% to the letter. She cut out the food she was sensitive to, had infrared saunas, as advised, and used the essential oils recommended.

After working with me, Litza reported how much her skin had improved and how she now had much more confidence.

She has also gone on to marry her partner and started a family. Happy days!

THE OUTSIDE-IN DETOX

'Up to 5,000 different chemicals are used in a number of scented products, many of which have never been tested for human safety.'

Nancy Lee Swanson, et al.[255]

This chapter shows how to avoid increasing your toxic load by reducing—and ideally, eliminating—toxins from your environment. Reducing your toxic load reduces the stress on your detoxification organs, including your skin. The less stress you put on your skin to detoxify your body, the greater chance you have of preventing blocked pores and breakouts.

There are so many environmental toxins to be aware of these days. Not only will I show you what they are, but I will also show you how to avoid them, as well as safe alternatives.

Common environmental toxins include:

- food
- tap water
- air pollution

---

[255] In Miller and Ashburn (1990).

- metal fillings and root canals
- personal care products/toiletries
- cosmetics
- perfumes, colognes and aftershaves
- cookware
- household cleaners
- household toxins
- car toxins (furnishings, A/C, etc.)
- prescription and non-prescription pharmaceuticals
- electromagnetic fields
- mental/emotional stress

Before you are overwhelmed, don't worry—just take everything one step at a time. Complete each of these tasks one at a time in your own time. Some people are able to take all of the recommendations on board at once, whilst others take a little longer. Go at the pace with which you are comfortable; however, be sure to remember that the quicker you are able to put these things into practice, the quicker you'll start to see clearer skin.

We pretty much covered food and water in the previous chapter, so I won't focus on them in this chapter, even though they play a crucial role in detoxification.

Air Pollution

Whether it is due to cigarette smoke, car fumes, industrial pollution or geoengineering, the air we breathe is full of toxins and contaminants these days. Whilst it would not be sensible for me to suggest you refrain from breathing, there are some things you can do to optimise the air you breathe.

Cigarette Smoke

The most obvious thing to suggest is that if you are a smoker, give up smoking. The amount of toxins you breathe in while smoking is truly astounding. Cigarettes give off over 4,000 chemicals, many of them toxic and/or carcinogenic (cancer-causing). Carbon monoxide, nitrogen oxides, hydrogen cyanide and ammonia are all present in cigarette smoke, along with 43 known carcinogens. Having never been a smoker, I cannot truly relate to the difficulties involved in giving up smoking. The closest I come to being able to sympathise is when I had eczema and had to give up the urge to scratch—no matter what I did, even though I knew that scratching would hurt and make me bleed, I still had the urge to scratch.

If you're not a smoker but are exposed to passive smoke, come up with solutions to avoid or at least minimise the smoke. Luckily, it is now illegal to smoke in many places around the world.

If someone in your home smokes, ask them to smoke outside. Even better, give them all the support they need to quit.

Car and Industrial Fumes

Car and industrial fumes (including geoengineering) are everywhere these days. If you live in a city or near an industrial site, you will likely get the worst of the toxic fumes. Whether from carbon monoxide, nitrogen oxide, sulfur dioxide, particulate emissions, lead, nanonised aluminium, nuclear fallout or any of the other major contaminants in our air, this is challenging to avoid.

One solution is to move to a rural area if you are able as the air, in general, is a little cleaner. However, there are few places on earth you can breathe clean air these days. If you can't move home, then do not despair, as there are still a few things you can do.

1. Try to get to a park (with a lot of trees) or to a clean beach every day for 20 to 30 minutes and take a gentle (or brisk) walk to breathe in cleaner air. Most large cities have large park areas like Central Park in New York or Hyde Park in London.

2. Use an air purifier at home and at work if possible.

3. Use D-Toxol and L-Glycine, supplements specifically formulated by a colleague of mine, Dr David Vaughan, to help off-
set environmental contamination. The supplement D-Toxol
should be taken with L-Glycine with meals. Dr Vaughan suggests taking two capsules of D-Toxol with one gram of L-Glycine with meals.

Supplement suppliers can be found at
https://eliminateadultacne.com/resources

Metal Dental Fillings and Root Canals

Metal Dental Fillings

Amalgam 'silver' fillings are comprised of *mercury*, a toxic heavy metal,
along with other toxic metals. Many researchers believe the mercury
leaches out of fillings over time and deposits in vital tissues in the body,
potentially causing a host of health problems.

Interestingly, my acne started at exactly the same time I started having metal fillings. Whether or not it prompted my acne, I can never
be sure. However, I do believe this is true in my adult life—because
the mercury is likely to have slowly poisoned me, it would stress my
immune system, causing long-term inflammation. The weakening of
my immune system would have left me more susceptible to infection.
As acne is potentially an infection, my body wasn't able to shake it off
effectively.

Most experts, including Dr Lawrence Wilson, recommend having
fillings containing mercury replaced as soon as possible. However, as
is the case with any profession, there are good and bad practitioners.
Many dentists today aren't trained to remove mercury safely, even if
they think they are. Because of this, it is advisable to use a biological or
holistic dentist specialising in safe mercury removal.

Details of how to prepare for a heavy metal detox are shown in
Chapter 8.

I have included an Amalgam Removal Dental Protocol to give you an idea of what to expect from a biological dentist at https://eliminateadultacne.com/resources

Root Canals

Despite being performed regularly by dentists, root canals were found ineffective at eradicating tooth infections almost 100 years ago by Weston A. Price, a research dentist with the American Dental Association and author of Nutrition and Physical Degeneration. After studying thousands of animals during his research, Price found the animals still had infections in their treated teeth that were leaching toxins into their bloodstreams. This means that if you have root canals, you may have infections in your mouth, leaching toxins into the rest of your body. For this reason, it is suggested you visit a biological or holistic dentist for advice and possible treatment.

If your body is overrun with toxins, and your organs of detoxification are unable to deal with them effectively, your skin may end up as the only place they can be excreted from your body, leading to breakouts.

Personal Care Products/Toiletries

Paul Chek, founder of The CHEK Institute, suggests, 'If it's on your skin, you're drinking it.' By saying this, he means that because our skin is semi-permeable, whatever we put on our skin enters our bloodstreams, and if it is poisonous, it has to be processed by our livers and is likely to be attacked by our immune systems, thus causing inflammation. Unfortunately, today's products are full of toxins and dangerous ingredients, according to many experts.

It is beyond the scope of this book to teach you everything about all toxic ingredients and the potential problems they cause. Instead, I suggest you type in the name of each product (or the ingredients of the products) you use into EWG's Skin Deep Cosmetics Database.[256] This

---

[256] 'Your guide,' n.d.

site independently checks the ingredients in products and their safety and gives a score for each product. The lower the score, the safer and healthier the product is. The EWG database is a great resource for finding out how healthy or harmful your products are and what might be a better alternative for you. If any of your products score higher than a two, I suggest that you might greatly benefit by swapping it for a less harmful product.

I have also listed some recommended personal care brands at https://eliminateadultacne.com/resources.

Cosmetics

Just like personal care products and toiletries, if the cosmetics are on your skin, you're drinking them. Also, like personal care products, many cosmetic products contain toxic ingredients that enter the bloodstream, and your detoxification organs must process the toxins.

Again, I suggest that you take your products and type each ingredient into EWG's Skin Deep Cosmetics Database to see how safe (or not) your products are.

Perfumes, Colognes and Aftershaves

As with personal care products and cosmetics, perfumes, colognes and aftershaves enter the bloodstream through the skin, and any toxic ingredients must be processed by the liver and other detoxification organs. There are, however, better alternatives you can use to smell nice, and some can even improve your health and skin.

Firstly, consider an organic, natural fragrance; there are a number of brands to choose from. You can also use organic essential oils, whether single oils, pre-blended oils, or blending your own. You do have to be careful with oils as many are produced cheaply and poorly, and the oils are often rancid. According to the *Essential Oils Desk Reference* compiled by Essential Science Publishing,[257] the following essential oils can help with acne:

- tea tree
- geranium
- lavender
- German or Roman chamomile
- rosewood
- cedarwood
- eucalyptus
- orange
- clove

At the time of writing this book, brands respected for their high quality include Essential Oil Wizardry and Du Terra.

Cookware

Many toxic chemicals are unfortunately used in cookware today. These toxins wouldn't be a problem if they didn't leach into the food, but under high heat and with the scraping of the cookware, the chemicals do leach into the food. Because most people eat at least three times per day, the toxic load is continuous every day. Chemicals such as plastic, aluminium, copper, cast iron, and in particular, chemicals in non-stick cookware, are toxic.

The following recommendations are better alternatives that might help when reducing your toxic load and improving your complexion:

- glass
- ceramic
- titanium

---

[257] 2000

Some good brands of cookware are Salad Master, Pyrex and Le Creuset. I recommend buying one new product a month or every other month unless you have a limitless budget. I don't want you to be so stressed financially that it reduces your gut permeability, thereby affecting your skin.

Household Cleaners

Many chemicals in most household cleaners contain toxins that your body's detoxification organs, including your skin, have to deal with. Some of the better brands of household cleaners of which I am aware include EcoZone and Ecover, as their ingredients are biodegradable and contain much fewer toxic ingredients.

Household Toxins

Today's homes are also full of toxins, including carpets, paint, vacuum cleaners, air fresheners, dust, mould and air conditioning units. My general advice would be to do your research before buying things for the home. Instead of carpets, laminated flooring is slightly less toxic. Use organic paints which are without Petro-chemicals. Cyclone vacuum cleaners give off less dust, and if you have an air conditioning unit, ensure it and the filters are regularly maintained. In addition, as I've mentioned before, good-quality air filters and water filtration systems are highly recommended.

Instead of using commercial air fresheners, which are highly toxic, use essential oils and diffuse the oils into your rooms. Diffusers are widely available and inexpensive.

Indoor plants are particularly good for removing pollutants from the home. The plants listed below are known to remove household pollutants:

- English ivy
- peace lily
- spider plant
- chrysanthemum
- mother-in-law's tongue

- golden pathos
- Madagascar dragon tree
- Waneckii
- heart leaf
- corn plant
- Chinese evergreen

If you live in a humid climate or home, I suggest having a dehumidifier, and if so, allow it to run all day in the winter. A moist home increases the likelihood of moulds and dust mites. You can also purchase test kits to test your home for moulds.

I interviewed Tim Swackhammer of Mold Medics in Episode 25 of my Podcast, *The Radical Health Rebel* (available on all major podcast platforms), where he discussed the dangers of mould in the home, how to prevent it and how best to deal with it safely.

Car Toxins

It's not just the pollution coming from car exhausts we need to be concerned about. The furnishings and components making up the insides of cars are also of concern. Chemicals such as cadmium, chlorine, lead, arsenic, bromine, mercury and tin are found in cars. As a rule of thumb, the newer the car, the higher the levels of chemicals. Hence, I tend to buy cars when they are at least three years old after most of the chemical outgassing has occurred.

My recommendation is to avoid the temptation to purchase a new car and avoid using car air fresheners. Use organic essential oils instead. Have your car cleaned inside and out regularly, using biodegradable cleaning products and a cyclone vacuum cleaner.

Prescription and Non-prescription Drugs

I must preface this section by stating that I am not a medical doctor, nor do I give advice when it comes to medication. Medication should only ever be taken on the advice of—and in consultation with—your medical doctor.

I do, however, suggest that prior to visiting your doctor, you educate yourself about the possible risks and benefits of your medication. If you have any concerns about a medical or recreational drug, you should discuss them openly with your doctor. It is also important to be aware that all medical drugs are toxic and known to cause side effects. Am I suggesting that medical drugs are bad? No. Medical drugs are fantastic for saving people's lives. Indeed, I wouldn't have survived beyond six weeks old without them.

However, in my own clinical experience, I have seen medications prescribed to people with chronic (non-life threatening) conditions when there are more natural, safer and effective non-drug options. The fact that medical drugs are toxic only serves to increase the amount of work required by your detoxification organs, including your skin, which could increase your likelihood of a breakout. It is also wise to educate yourself on any potential side effects that a medical drug may cause. This is very easy to do at the Drugs.com[258] website.

If you use recreational drugs like heroin, cocaine, MDMA (Ecstasy), LCD (Acid) or marijuana, know that these are not controlled substances (in most countries), and apart from the active ingredients, they are nearly always mixed with many unknown compounds that can be highly toxic and dangerous. Marijuana is known to have a high level of heavy metals like mercury, depending on the soil in which it is grown. Whether marijuana is legal or not where you live, be sure that if you use it, it was grown in the cleanest of soils.

It will help you detoxify if you are able to stop using recreational drugs; however, you might wish to receive professional help or advice before doing so.

Ultimately, the healthier you are, the fewer drugs you need to take, whether medical or recreational. Following the tips in this book will improve your health if followed stringently and consistently, reducing your requirements for medical drugs in most circumstances.

---

[258] 'Find Drugs,' n.d.

Electromagnetic Fields

In the modern world, electromagnetic fields (EMFs) are all around us, and it's almost impossible to avoid them.

Common sources of EMFs include:

- televisions
- mobile phones
- mobile phone masts
- Wi-Fi and Bluetooth
- computers
- electrical home appliances
- indoor lights
- power lines
- home wiring
- airport and military radar
- substations and transformers

Current research highlights more and more adverse effects on our health (I have over 200 references suggesting this is the case). Whilst EMFs may not directly cause acne, they may reduce the body's vitality and available nutrients and suppress the immune system, which might lead to acne.

Whilst moving to a desert island would be ideal, most of us live in an urban or suburban environment and can't avoid EMFs, but we can minimise them.

You can:

- measure EMFs both inside and outside your home;
- measure EMFs from appliances when they are operating and when they are turned off—some appliances (like TVs) still draw currents even when they are off;
- find the source of the EMFs around you;

- move furniture, particularly the bed and seating arrangements, away from areas of high electrical fields;

- don't sleep under an electric blanket or in a waterbed—if you insist on using these, unplug them before going to bed (don't just turn them off), as even though there is no magnetic field when they are turned off, there may still be a high electric field;

- don't sit too close to your TV set—distance yourself at least six feet away and use a meter to help you decide where it is safe to sit;

- rearrange your office and home area so that you are not exposed to EMFs from electric appliances and computers—at home, it is best to place all major electrical appliances (such as computers, TVs, refrigerators, etc.) against outside walls so you don't create an EMF field in the adjoining room;

- don't sit too close to your computer—computer monitors vary greatly in the strength of their EMFs, so be sure to check yours with a meter;

- don't stand close to your microwave oven if you have one—better still, dispose of it safely—as even when they are plugged in and switched off, they give off large amounts of EMFs;

- never have your mobile phone near you when it is switched on—ensure it is in aeroplane mode and Bluetooth is switched off whenever it is near you and only switch aeroplane mode off when using the phone;

- never hold your mobile phone to your head—always use the speaker or air tubes;

- never have your mobile phone switched on when in a car or train, as the metal surroundings trap radio waves inside the vehicle;

- avoid going near power lines, transformers, radar domes and microwave towers;

- move all electrical appliances at least six feet from your bed, and eliminate wires running under or near your bed;

- eliminate dimmers and three-way switches;
- be wary of cordless appliances such as electric toothbrushes and razors;
- choose not to wear a quartz-analogue watch because it radiates pulsating EMFs along your acupuncture meridians (so-called smart watches are much worse!); use older mechanical windup watches as a safer alternative;
- wear as little jewellery as possible and take it off at night;
- remember that EMFs pass right through walls, so the EMF on your meter could be radiating from the next room or your neighbours;
- bear in mind that items used close to the body emit EMFs (hair dryers, for instance, produce high electrical fields, as do electric blankets, which are close to the body all night long—'electric under blankets and over blankets give off high magnetic fields that penetrate about 6 or 7 inches into the body;'[259]
- avoid the use of electrically operated adjustable beds and furniture as they give off strong magnetic fields;
- move electrical clocks and clock radios so they are at least one metre from your head and
- sit as far away as possible from computer screens and TVs as they are major sources of electrical fields, or use a device to neutralise the electrical fields.

There are a wide range of products available to protect you from electromagnetic stress. 'These include meters and monitors so that you can measure the fields, products for personal protection, products to protect you in your home or office'[260] and products to help clear the body of electromagnetic stress.

---

[259] Kingston, 2023
[260] 'Electrical Sensitivity,' 2014

You can find information on products to reduce EMR at
https://eliminateadultacne.com/resources.

Mental/Emotional Stress

In today's modern world, it is a real challenge to avoid mental and/or emotional stress. Whether it is financial stress, relationship stress, family stress, work deadlines or your overly demanding boss, we all seem to have stress. In Chapter 5, I described why excess stress is not ideal if you want to rid yourself of acne, so I won't repeat it here.

The number one recommendation I can make to reduce mental/emotional stress is to take time out each day to spend on your own in silence, also known as meditation. There are many different ways to do it, but as a simple guideline, spend ten minutes per day on your own, focusing on breathing in and out of your abdomen. As you breathe in, your abdomen should move outwards away from your spine, and as you breathe out, your abdomen should move inwards towards your spine.

In addition, write down a list of all the things you enjoy doing and a list of all the things you dislike doing. Each week, set aside time to do one thing you enjoy doing until it becomes part of your everyday life. Once that happens, choose one thing you dislike doing and work out a way you won't have to do it, perhaps by finding someone to do it for you. You might consider trading tasks with someone else or paying them in return.

Think seriously about things like your job, your relationship and so on and decide if they serve you well and make you happy. If not, decide the changes you need to make.

Other things discussed in this book—like being clear on your goals and core values, eating right for your Metabolic Type® and going to bed on time—will also help with your mental/emotional wellbeing, ultimately helping to improve your skin.

Chapter summary/Key takeaways

In summary:

- Environmental toxins are everywhere, and when inhaled, swallowed or absorbed into the body, they increase our toxic load, thereby increasing the requirements of detoxifying through the skin and reducing the amount of nutrients available to the skin, which increases the likelihood of acne.

- It is important to identify all potential environmental toxins in your environment.

- It is crucial to reduce, replace or eliminate as many environmental toxins as possible to reduce your toxic load and reduce the likelihood of acne.

In the next chapter, I discuss the inside-out detox.

SUCCESS STORY 5

Meet Esther.

Esther was in her forties when I met her through a friend. She had really bad breakouts and was very embarrassed about her skin. Her acne was so bad that even applying makeup couldn't conceal it, and she tried many different facials and cleaning routines without success.

Esther purchased the first edition of this book after chatting with me, and in a very short period of time, she improved her diet—especially reducing sugar and flour intake—and she noticed a great improvement very quickly, which greatly improved her confidence levels. She now uses much less makeup than before because she doesn't need to conceal her acne.

Suffice it to say, she was very pleased with the progress in a short period of time and looked forward to continued improvements and a further reduction in the frequency and severity of breakouts as she made her way through the book.

THE INSIDE-OUT DETOX

· ·

> 'Toxicity is a one-way street leading to disease.
>
> The key to healing the impossible is to reverse the toxicity...
>
> The most fascinating part is that once these chemicals are removed, conditions that have baffled the most prestigious medical centers [sic] and diseases that were thought to be incurable, magically melt away.'
>
> Sherry Rogers MD

In this chapter, I show you procedures to help detoxify your body from the inside out.

As already stated, the skin is an organ of detoxification. To avoid acne, we must, therefore, help other organs of detoxification by lowering our toxic loads. One way to lower your toxic load is to complete regular detox procedures. It is well known that performing some of these detox procedures can help quickly clear the skin.

Whenever I felt a breakout coming on, a coffee enema once a day for three days normally kept them at bay.

Many of these 'cleanses' have been adapted from studying with William Wolcott, the author of The Metabolic Typing Diet[261] and the world's leading authority on Metabolic Typing®.

To me, cleanses are similar to having your car serviced. Your car needs a regular change of oil and spark plugs to keep it in good working order. In this day and age, our bodies need regular detoxing to help reduce the poisoning of the cells, the disruption of enzyme reactions and the displacement of necessary nutrients and to reduce the stockpiling of toxins in vital organs.

It is not recommended that you use any of the cleanses below if you are not following the correct diet for your Metabolic Type®, as it would be like trying to build a house in a known earthquake zone without first building a solid foundation.

There are a series of cleanses effective at helping eliminate toxins from the body, thereby reducing acne. They are:

- infrared saunas
- coffee enemas
- colon cleanses
- castor oil packs
- liver/gallbladder flushes
- cell cleanses
- skin cleanses

PRIOR TO PERFORMING CLEANSES, IT IS RECOMMENDED YOU GAIN APPROVAL FROM YOUR DOCTOR.

The other cleanses you may do were discussed in Chapter 6 on the Gut-Skin Axis.

---

[261] 2002

Infrared Sauna

This section explains why infrared saunas are beneficial for acne sufferers, where you can find or buy them, when to do them, and how best to do them.

How Do Infrared Saunas Work?

Infrared (IR) saunas help to gently detoxify heavy metals and other toxic substances through the action of sweating caused by the heat of IR lamps. IR saunas also enhance circulation and increase the oxidation of tissues. The increase of heat helps decongest internal organs via blood flow to the skin.

IR saunas also help stimulate the parasympathetic nervous system, allowing you to relax. The sympathetic nervous system is activated when you are stressed, which, as you may remember, is not a good idea if you want great skin.

It is believed IR saunas remove toxins much quicker than conventional saunas.

What Items Will I Need?

- buy or build your own IR sauna for your home or
- find a facility where you can go to have IR saunas.

When To Do Them:

- Every day or as often as possible for the first six months and weekly at the very least.

How To Have an Infrared Sauna:

1. **Receive approval from your doctor first–IMPORTANT! This is especially true if you have a diagnosed condition or are taking medication. ALL saunas should be avoided if you're pregnant!**

2. Do NOT exercise or have a big meal within two hours of having a sauna.

3. Preheat the sauna to approximately 100°F (40°C).

4. Drink two glasses of water before the session.

5. Begin taking IR saunas for 20 minutes each time. After a few weeks, you may slowly increase to 30 or 40 minutes. Increasing session time too soon may lead to unpleasant healing reactions that can be dangerous, so tread carefully!!!

6. Wear as little as possible so the heat penetrates the skin. Wearing more than a bathing suit will greatly reduce the effects.

7. Stop the session and leave the sauna if you feel faint, stop sweating, or your heart starts to race.

8. After the sauna, take a warm shower using only good-quality skin cleansing products, as discussed in Chapter 9.

9. Relax for 10-15 minutes following a sauna to allow the body to re-adjust. Do not go straight back to everyday duties.

10. IR saunas are best used first thing in the morning or last thing at night, when you are the most relaxed, which will allow you to sweat more.

11. Pregnant women and young children should not use saunas.

12. It might be prudent to have someone with you when you first start taking saunas.

Details of where you can find commercial infrared saunas, build your own or purchase them can be found on the resources page of my website at

https://eliminateadultacne.com/resources.

Coffee Enemas

This section explains why coffee enemas are beneficial for acne sufferers, what items you will need, when to do them, and how to do them.

How Do Enemas Work?

Coffee enemas aid the liver in the detoxification process and the colon in eliminating its contents. The efficient removal of toxins and metabolic waste is crucial if you want to minimise the likelihood of breakouts.

What Items Will I Need?

You will need the following items:

1	YOUR DOCTOR'S PERMISSION!
2	organic coffee
3	pure water
4	coffee grinder
5	coffee maker (optional)
6	enema bucket or enema bag
7	enema tube
8	natural lubricant (herbal lubricant, butter, coconut oil)

When To Do Them:

- every other day for the first four months
- whenever required after that or if you feel a breakout coming on
- leading up to big events to help avoid breakouts on or just before the big day if you choose to do so

How To Do a Coffee Enema:

1. Receive approval from your doctor.
2. Gather all the items listed above.
3. Put a teaspoon or two of fresh organic coffee beans into a coffee grinder.
4. Grind the coffee beans.

5. Place the coffee into a coffee maker or saucepan with one litre of pure water (not tap water).

   a. Use between ½ and two teaspoons of coffee (start with less, you can always add more).

6. Whilst the water is heating up, place the enema tube on the enema bucket or enema bag and close the clip.

7. Once boiled, pour the coffee into the enema bucket or bag.

8. Allow the coffee to cool down to room temperature (or add cold water).

9. Whilst the coffee is cooling, lay some towels on the floor in your bathroom, close to your toilet. You might also want something to rest your head on.

10. You will need to use something to put the enema bucket on or a place to hang your enema bag when ready.

11. You might also want to put on some relaxing music.

12. Once the enema is at room temperature, hold the enema bucket or bag over your bath, shower or toilet, open the clip on the tube and allow some coffee to flow out. Quickly close the clip.

13. Place the bucket or bag somewhere higher than the floor (as gravity will be required for the coffee to flow).

14. Take the natural lubricant and smear it on the end of the tube, ensuring you lubricate the holes.

15. Lie on the towels on your left side and get as comfortable as possible.

16. Slowly—very slowly—insert the end of the tube into your anus. Exhale and relax as you gently push in the tube. Keep pushing it in until it won't go any farther.

17. Once it is in, let out some coffee by opening the clip on the enema tube. As long as there isn't any air in the tube and the

bucket or bag is above the height of the ground by at least 12 inches (25cm), it should flow easily.

18. Start by releasing a small amount, then, when you feel confident and comfortable, slowly allow more coffee in until the bucket or bag is empty.

19. You can close the clip on the tube, or you can leave it open.

    a. Leaving the clip closed prevents any coffee from going back up into the bucket or bag.

    b. Leaving the clip open allows gas to be released.

20. As you lie there, massage the left side of your abdomen between your ribs and your pelvis (this is where your descending colon is located).

21. If you feel painful gas, try to relax, breathe, and let it pass, but do not retain the coffee if it gets too uncomfortable.

22. If you are unable to retain the coffee, it may be due to:

    a. too much coffee in the solution

    b. water too hot or too cold

    c. too much water

    d. excessive gas

    It may require trying less coffee, using a different water temperature or using less water. It may also improve with each enema you do.

23. After five minutes on your left side, move to lie on your back. Massage from right to left just under your rib cage (this is where your transverse colon is located) as you go.

24. Again, if you feel painful gas, try to relax, breathe and let it pass, but do not retain the coffee if it gets too uncomfortable.

25. After five minutes on your back, turn to lie on your right side.

26. Massage the right side of your abdomen between your ribs and pelvis (this is where your ascending colon is located).

27. Again, if you feel painful gas, try to relax, breathe and let it pass, but do not retain the coffee if it gets too uncomfortable.

28. Once you are finished, slowly get up to standing, pick up the bucket or bag, sit on the toilet and gently remove the tube.

29. Once you have removed the tube, allow your bowels to evacuate their contents into the toilet. Remember that a lot of it is water, so be patient when allowing it time to come out. It may take a few minutes.

Details of where you can purchase the items required for coffee enemas can be found on the resources page of our website at http://www.eliminateadultacne.com/resources.

Detox Protocol for Metal Filling Removal

If you are going to have metal fillings or root canals removed by a well-skilled biological or holistic dentist, it is advised to use following the protocol to minimise any ingestion of the metal being removed.

Add the following to your protocol starting a couple of weeks before the removal:

1. HMD protocol plus chlorella. Also, have HMD Lavage available for the day of the procedure.

2. On the day of removal, take a 'large' (20 caps) amount of chlorella, but no vitamin C until after removal. Rinse your mouth immediately with HMD Lavage.

3. Immediately after removal, take 4,000 mg of vitamin C. The dentist will sometimes offer you intravenous vitamin C directly afterwards.

4. Continue with the HMD at a regular dosage for a week after the procedure.

Details of products for heavy metal detoxification can be found at http://www.eliminateadultacne.com/resources.

Colon Cleanse

This section explains why colon cleanses may be beneficial for reducing acne, what items you will need, when to do them, and how to do them.

How Do Colon Cleanses Work?

There are many different colon cleanses available, but most involve drinking a gelatinous and bulky mixture containing psyllium husks, herbs and water throughout the day in large quantities along with large quantities of water.

Colon cleanses generally include either a reduction of food (particularly animal-based foods). Some may choose to fast during the cleanse, which lasts from three to five days.

Once consumed, the mixture sticks to the lining of the colon, soaking into any hardened encrusted material to soften it. This can be sloughed away with the help of coffee enemas and massaging of the colon, unblocking the colon, and removing the toxic material.

As I've said before, the efficient removal of toxins and metabolic waste is crucial if you want to minimise your likelihood of breakouts.

What Items Will I Need?

There are many different brands and products on the market. The ones I use are easily attainable, and they are listed below.

You will need the following items:

1	YOUR DOCTOR'S PERMISSION!!!
2	Everything required for coffee enemas (see above)
3	Puritox-200 (to make liquid Bentonite)
4	pure water (not tap water)
5	a pint (1/2 litre) jar

6	LBF#1 (LBF = Lower Bowel Formula)
7	LBF#2 (LBF = Lower Bowel Formula)
8	fresh organic vegetables (to juice)
9	a vegetable juicer
10	multi-vitamins for your Metabolic Type®
11	Ultra-Greens

When To Do Them:

- Every three months.

How To Do a Colon Cleanse:

1. For at least seven days, take the LBF#1 formula to ensure you have one to two bowel movements every day. The LBF#1 formula can be taken with meals and/or before bed.

   a. Dosages will vary from person to person. Start with one per day and increase as necessary.

2. After seven days of having at least one bowel movement a day, complete the following:

   a. Upon awakening, drink ½ cup of liquid Bentonite (Puritox-200 in water).

   b. Follow with one to two glasses of water.

3. Then, every three hours (five times per day for three to five days), make and drink the following mixture:

   a. add one cup of pure water into a pint jar

   b. add one tablespoon of liquid Bentonite

   c. add one tablespoon of LBF#2

   d. screw on the lid and shake vigorously for 15 seconds

   e. chug down the solution as quickly as possible

   f. follow with at least three cups of water.

4. In between mixtures, drink as much pure water and/or freshly juiced vegetable juice as required.

5. Do not take your usual supplements except for Synergy Com and Ultra Greens (right for your Metabolic Type®)

6. Eat as little as possible (to give your digestive system and colon a rest) with an emphasis on fresh organic vegetables and fruit. If possible, have fresh juice, Synergy Com and Ultra Greens instead of meals.

7. If you need food, do not starve yourself, especially if you get light-headed. Just eat as small an amount as you can get away with. Please note that this is not recommended for more than a few days!

8. Take a coffee enema in the afternoon each day. Using just one cup of coffee at a time, massage a small area, starting on the lower left area of your abdomen. Massage any hardened areas until soft, then add more coffee and continue around the colon. The enema may take up to one hour.

   a. Most people tend to take a Friday off work so they can eat lightly and complete the coffee enemas on a Friday, Saturday, and Sunday. It isn't suggested to try to live a normal life whilst doing a colon cleanse, just like you wouldn't drive your car when it's in for a service.

9. You can return to normal eating and your normal lifestyle after three days. However, you may need to take the mixture first thing in the morning and last thing at night to add bulk to your stools until normal healthy bowel function returns.

Details of where you can purchase the items required for colon cleanses can be found on the resources page of our website at http://www.eliminateadultacne.com/resources.

Example of A Colon Cleanse Daily Schedule:

Upon Awakening	drink ½ cup (0.12 litre) of liquid Bentonite followed by one to two glasses of water
08:00	light BREAKFAST or fresh juice and Ultra Green
08:45	water (mineral or reverse osmosis), minimum of one glass
09:30	first mixture
10:15	water (mineral or reverse osmosis), minimum of one glass
11:00	light LUNCH or fresh juice and Ultra Green
11:45	water (mineral or reverse osmosis), minimum of one glass
12:30	second mixture
13:15	water (mineral or reverse osmosis), minimum of one glass
14:00	fresh juice and Ultra Green
14:45	water (mineral or reverse osmosis), minimum of one glass
15:30	third mixture
16:45	water (mineral or reverse osmosis), minimum of one glass
17:00	light dinner or fresh juice and Ultra Green
17:45	water (mineral or reverse osmosis), minimum of one glass
18:30	fourth mixture
19:15	water (mineral or reverse osmosis), minimum of one glass
20:00	fresh juice and Ultra Green
20:45	water (mineral or reverse osmosis), minimum of one glass
21:30	fifth mixture
22:15	take LBF#1 capsules before bed

*See Point 3 above on how to make the mixture

Castor Oil Packs

This section explains why castor oil packs are beneficial for acne sufferers, what items you will need, when to do them, and how to do them.

How Do Castor Oil Packs Work?

Castor oil packs were used by many ancient societies for their health benefits. Today, castor oil packs are still used for their many different benefits. In the case of acne, castor oil packs can be used to help detoxify the liver and other tissues and improve elimination and the stimulation of the liver and gallbladder.

What Items Will I Need?

You will need:

1	100% pure, cold-pressed castor oil.
2	wool flannel (not cotton)
3	heating pad or hot water bottle
4	plastic wrap/Saran Wrap/cling film
5	oven
6	baking dish

When To Do Them:

- Following your doctor's approval.
- Whenever you desire.
- The five days leading up to a liver/gallbladder cleanse.

How To Do a Castor Oil Pack:

1. Put your oven on low heat.
2. Take the wool flannel and fold it into three or four layers.
3. Soak the flannel in castor oil.

4. Place the soaked flannel in a baking dish.

5. Place the baking dish in the oven.

6. Monitor the flannel in the oven to ensure it doesn't get too hot and catch fire.

7. Warm the flannel to a heat where it won't be too hot to place on your skin.

8. Once adequately heated, remove from the oven (remember to turn your oven off).

9. Take a length of plastic wrap approximately 15 inches (30cm) long.

10. Lie down somewhere comfortable, like your sofa.

11. Rub a liberal amount of castor oil over the area of your upper right abdomen, just under the ribs.

12. Place the warmed flannel over the same area.

13. Cover the flannel with plastic wrap.

14. Place a heating pad or hot water bottle over the cling film.

    a. Note: heating pads normally give off a high level of EMFs. For this reason, I prefer a hot water bottle, even though they don't maintain heat as well. Having two hot water bottles and switching over as the heat dissipates from the one being used is one option for maintaining optimal heat levels.

15. Relax for 60 minutes.

16. Remove when finished. Wash the affected skin.

17. Keep the wool flannel in a sealed container or bag. Clean the flannel if it becomes discoloured other than the colour of the oil. The discolouration will be due to the toxins being released, and you don't want to add them back in!

Details of where you can purchase the items required for Castor Oil Packs can be found on the resources page of our website at https://eliminateadultacne.com/resources.

Liver/Gallbladder Flush

In this section, I explain why liver/gallbladder flushes are beneficial for acne sufferers, what items you will need, when to do them, and how to do them.

How Do Liver/Gallbladder Flushes Work?

The flushes work by aiding the body's natural process of keeping bile flowing, thereby helping to minimise any debris building up in the gallbladder. The flush helps expel any substances held in the liver and gallbladder, such as toxins, stones and pre-stone sludge, including stagnant bile, calcium, cholesterol and toxins. By maintaining the natural detoxification pathway, you reduce the likelihood of any toxins backing up in the system and trying to escape through the skin, causing acne.

What Items Will I Need?

You will need:

1	Ultra-Phos Drops
2	malic acid tablets
3	mag citrate or Epsom salts
4	organic cold-pressed olive oil
5	fresh ginger
6	HCL tablets (HCL)
7	fresh organic apples, oranges and/or grapefruit
8	fresh fruit and whipping cream
9	Castor Oil Pack (see section above)
10	coffee enema equipment (see section above)

When To Do Them:

- following your doctor's approval
- every three months, following a colon cleanse

How To Do a Liver/Gallbladder Flush:

1. Continue the Acne Elimination Diet as normal.

2. Take three Malic acid tablets four times per day (with or without food).

3. You may wish to drink as much freshly pressed carrot juice as long as your doctor does not suggest otherwise due to blood sugar problems or if it makes you feel uncomfortable, worsens your acne or if you have a sensitivity to carrots.

    a. Only use organic carrots, ideally freshly squeezed in a juicer.

    b. Do not use store-bought pasteurised juice.

4. Add a total of 90 drops of Ultra-Phos to the carrot juice or any other juice each day.

5. Do a Castor Oil Pack (see above) over the right side of your abdomen, just under the rib cage, one hour before bed or at any other convenient time of the day.

6. Complete the above for five days.

7. On day six, eat a normal breakfast and lunch with your appropriate supplements.

8. Two hours after lunch, dissolve two tablespoons of Mag-Citrate or Epsom salts in ½ a cup of warm, pure water and drink it.

    a. If the taste is unbearable, you can chase it with a little citrus juice.

9. Four hours after lunch, have a coffee enema (see above) with ¼ cup of Mag-Citrate or Epsom salts dissolved into it.

10. Five hours after lunch, dissolve one tablespoon of Mag-Citrate or Epsom salts in ½ cup of warm, pure water and drink it.

11. Six hours after lunch, either fast (abstain from food) or eat a fruit and whipped cream salad made with a variety of fresh fruit with an emphasis on the cream.

12. Just before bed, drink ½ cup of extra virgin olive oil.

    a. Add an equal amount of organic grapefruit or diluted lemon juice to the oil if you choose.

    b. Alternatively, alternate sips of oils and sips of juice until the oil is finished.

    c. Due to the release of toxins, you may feel nauseous. Adding one or two HCL tablets and some freshly grated ginger to the juice should help.

    d. Having a coffee enema and ¼ cup of Epsom salts can usually halt nausea. This should be prepared prior to taking the oil (and juice). If you have nausea during the night, having an immediate enema usually stops the nausea.

    e. Go to bed immediately after taking the oil. Lie on your right side with your knees drawn to your chest.

    f. The next morning, have another coffee enema with ¼ cup of Mag-Citrate or Epsom salts dissolved in it and drink ½ cup of water with one tablespoon of Mag-Citrate or Epsom salts dissolved into it.

    g. Resume the Acne Elimination Diet the next day, but eat lightly for breakfast and lunch, minimising animal proteins, fats, and oils.

Possible Reactions from a Liver/Gallbladder Flush
The morning after the cleanse, you might observe greenish matter in your stool (faeces), which can be soft or hard and stone-like. The greenish matter—mostly composed of coagulated bile from the gallbladder or liver if the gallbladder has been removed—may show up for several days following the cleanse. This normally suggests a successful cleanse.

Most people have no adverse reactions, but as stated above, some may feel mild, temporary nausea due to the elimination of toxins. My own experience has been that with each subsequent cleanse, the level of nausea is reduced (as the level of toxins being released is reduced). A common reaction following a cleanse is a general feeling of wellbeing, more energy and better skin.

> Details of where you can purchase the items required for liver/ gallbladder flushes can be found at https://eliminateadultacne.com/resources.

Cell Cleanse

In this section, I explain why cell cleanses are beneficial for acne sufferers, what items you will need, when to do them, and how to do them.

How Do Cell Cleanses Work?

As I am sure you've gathered by now, toxins increase the likelihood of acne. Therefore, it is important to reduce the levels of toxins in the body—creating an acidic environment—at every opportunity. Cell cleanses help detoxify by alkalising the bloodstream along with all bodily systems. It is believed the alkalising effect helps open cell membranes, allowing toxins to be released.

The regular intake of water is also believed to help release toxins and regulate blood sugar and mineral balance.

What Items Will I Need?

You will need:

1	Mag-Citrate or Epsom salts
2	pure water
3	6 grapefruits
4	6 lemons
5	12 oranges

6	a 1 gallon (3.8 litre) container
7	potatoes
8	carrots
9	beets (beetroot)
10	onions
11	garlic
12	celery
13	dark greens
14	sieve
15	coffee enema equipment (see section above)
16	organic, unprocessed sea salt

When To Do Them:

- Following the go-ahead from your doctor.
- Twice per year.

How To Do a Cell Cleanse:

1. Prepare an alkaline punch:
   a. Combine the juice of six grapefruits, six lemons and twelve oranges in a gallon (3.8 litre) container. Fill the rest of the container with purified water.

2. Prepare a potassium broth:
   a. Fill a pot with 25% each of organic:
      i. potato peelings
      ii. carrot peelings and chopped beets
      iii. chopped onion and garlic
      iv. chopped celery and dark greens

b. Cover with purified water and simmer for one to four hours.

c. Strain and discard vegetables.

3. On Day 1:

a. Do a coffee enema upon awakening.

b. Take one tablespoon of Mag Citrate (or Epsom salts) dissolved in ½ cup (0.12 litre) of warm water 30 minutes later.

c. Take one more tablespoon of Mag Citrate (or Epsom salts) dissolved in ½ cup (0.12 litre) of warm water 30 minutes later.

d. Take one more tablespoon of Mag Citrate (or Epsom salts) dissolved in ½ cup (0.12 litre) of warm water again 30 minutes later.

e. Drink four swallows of the alkaline punch two hours later.

f. Drink four more swallows of the alkaline punch 30 minutes later.

g. Drink four more swallows of the alkaline punch or plain water 30 minutes later, repeating every 30 minutes thereafter for the next five hours.

h. Do not take any supplements on this day.

4. Day 2:

a. Drink two swallows of pure water every 30 minutes over an eight-hour period.

b. Freely consume fresh carrot juice and potassium broth as your appetite dictates. You can add organic sea salt to the broth to taste.

c. Complete one or two coffee enemas during the day.

d. Minimise activities and rest as much as possible.

e. Do not take any supplements.

5. Day 3:

a. Resume your usual diet and supplement regime.

<u>Possible Reactions from a Cell Cleanse</u>
No adverse reactions are likely.

> Details of where you can purchase the items required for cell cleanses can be found on the resources page of our website at https://eliminateadultacne.com /resources.

Chapter summary/Key takeaways

- Using infrared saunas and cleansing protocols can help eliminate toxins from the body.
- Before performing any detoxes, obtain approval from your doctor, especially if you have a diagnosed medical condition.
- There are a series of detoxes and cleanses you can perform to eliminate toxins from your body, thereby reducing your likelihood of acne.

In the next chapter, I show you a daily skin-cleansing protocol.

SUCCESS STORY 6

Meet Leah.

Leah was a 27-year-old who worked in insurance. Leah hadn't ever made much of an effort to eat healthily, and she loved chocolate. Before the age of 27, she ate 'whatever she wanted', and she had maintained a very healthy figure and completely clear skin. It was a big shock to her when she broke out for the first time in her life and just months away from her wedding. Leah was in a panic because she didn't want bad skin on her wedding day.

After testing, it was found that Leah had a minor dysbiosis and parasite infection that may or may not have been causing health issues (sometimes parasites can be present without causing problems).

I advised Leah on her nutrition and lifestyle and helped improve her gut microbiome. A few months in, there was some, but not much, improvement in Leah's skin, and she was in a state of panic.

At that point, I tested for heavy metals, and it turned out that Leah had very high levels of mercury in her blood. When explaining the potential causes, I mentioned that fish, especially tuna, has mercury in it. It turns out that Leah had eaten tuna for lunch every day for years. I advised Leah to use liposomal glutathione to help remove the mercury from the blood, and in a matter of weeks, Leah's skin was back to normal.

This is a good example of how this cause differed from the other examples in this book and how, in some situations, you need to keep going until you find the solution or combination of solutions that works for you. Remember that we are all different.

THE SKIN CLEANSING RITUAL

· ·

'If it's on your skin, you're drinking it.'

Paul Chek

In this chapter, I show you three skin cleansing techniques and a daily skin ritual to keep your skin in tip-top condition.

Skin Cleanse

In this section, I show you three techniques you can use to cleanse your skin.

How Do Skin Cleanses Work?

Skin cleanses work by:

- removing dead skin cells,
- cleansing the pores,
- stimulating hormone- and oil-producing glands in the skin,
- improving circulation,
- assisting with the removal of stored toxins, including metabolic waste, heavy metals, excess minerals and environmental con-taminants and
- restoring optimal pH levels of the skin.

What Items Will I Need?

1	Dry Skin Brushing:
	1. a natural bristle brush
2	Skin Rub:
	2. castor oil
	3. organic extra virgin olive oil
	4. container (to mix the oils)
	5. bath and shower
3	Vinegar Bath:
	6. organic apple cider vinegar
	7. bath and shower

When To Do Them:

1. Dry Skin Brushing: daily
2. Skin Rub: often
3. Vinegar Bath: often

How To Do a Skin Cleanse:

1. Dry Skin Brushing:

    a. Using a natural bristle brush, brush your skin first thing in the morning and last thing at night.

    b. Dry brush prior to bathing or showering.

    c. Using a circular motion, brush vigorously over the whole body.

    d. Start brushing from the head towards the heart, the hands towards the heart and then the toes towards the heart.

    e. Include the palms of the hands and the soles of the feet.

    f. Clean the brush every few days with soap and water.

2. Skin Rub:

   a. Dry brush the skin (as above).

   b. Mix equal parts of castor oil and olive oil in a container.

   c. Rub your skin from head to toe with the mixture, including your scalp, palms of the hands and soles of the feet.

   d. Keeping the mixture on, bathe in hot water for 15 minutes– **BE EXTRA CAREFUL GETTING INTO AND OUT OF THE BATH WITH THE OIL ON YOUR SKIN!!!**

      i. It is HIGHLY ADVISED to use a rubber mat in the bath to help prevent slipping!

   e. Following the bath, pat yourself dry with a towel, and go to bed for one hour under heavy covers.

   f. Take a shower. You may need to use a little baking soda to help get off the oil.

3. Vinegar Bath:

   a. Soak in a bath with two added cups (0.47 litres) of organic apple cider vinegar.

   b. Soak for a minimum of 20 minutes.

   c. Drain the bath and shower as usual.

Possible Reactions from a Skin Cleanse
No adverse reactions.

Details of where you can purchase the items required for skin cleanses can be found at https://eliminateadultacne.com /resources.

The Daily Skin Ritual

In this section, I show you how to cleanse your skin effectively to reduce the likelihood of acne and keep it look glowing and healthy, helping you to get your confidence back with abundance.

This chapter has purposely been placed towards the end of the book, as it is far less important in terms of reducing acne in the long term. However, it might be possible it's just what you need to add the icing on the cake, so to speak, ensuring your acne doesn't come back.

My clients' experience is that when they follow the Daily Skin Ritual, their skin is better, and it helps them avoid breakouts. As previously mentioned, acne can be caused by blockages in the hair follicles. So, if we keep the skin—and therefore, the hair follicles—clear, we may reduce the likelihood of acne.

The first thing to be clear about is the products you use to clean your skin. Find a good brand that does not use toxic chemicals, which may eventually increase your chance of acne. There are some good brands available, and you will find a list of them on the resources page of my website.

> For product recommendations, check out
> https://eliminateadultacne.com /resources.

Remember that your skin is porous, which means that whatever you put on your skin gets into your bloodstream, so if it is toxic, your liver will have to process the toxins. If your liver and other detoxification organs are already overburdened, the toxins may begin to escape through the skin, causing acne. A good rule to follow is that if it's not safe to eat or drink, it's not safe to put on your skin.

If you want to avoid poisoning yourself and potentially increasing your chance of acne or any other chronic degenerative disease, please check out EWG's Skin Deep site (URL in Resources) before buying any more personal care products and cosmetics. You can also check your own products on the site, too, in order to find out how safe—or how toxic—they are.

This routine is simple—simpler, in fact, than you might have imagined: only wash your face (chest and back) with clean, unchlorinated water (no soap). Whilst your skin is still moist, use organic aloe vera gel, with or without added tea tree oil, on your face and any skin with acne, or that has recently been exposed to the sun for any period of time. Not only is aloe vera cooling and moisturising, but it has an acidic pH, which, as you will remember from earlier in this book, is advantageous for skin and the skin microbiome. Aloe vera is also anti-inflammatory, aiding in wound healing, which is great for acne.

Restoring skin to an optimal acidic pH can also be achieved both with topical applications as well as oral supplementation, such as borage oil,[262, 263] and as mentioned above, organic aloe vera. [109]

If it seems strange not to use soap on your affected areas—it did to me when it was first suggested to me—trust in the process as my skin took another step forward in how good it looked, and you'll likely be surprised how water alone is surprisingly good at cleaning the skin.

Body Wash/Soap/Shower Gel

Ensure you use a good quality body wash or shower gel. Dr Julie Greenberg, a Holistic Dermatologist, suggests only washing your 'pits' (armpits) and 'bits' (crotch area). It is important to keep your skin in a slightly acidic state, and washing with soaps and body washes often leaves the skin alkaline, increasing the likelihood of acne.

Washing the rest of the body with unchlorinated (filtered) tap water is all you need. It is crucial to use either a whole-house water filter or a shower filter that filters out toxins, especially chlorine (which is basically bleach) and heavy metals.

Remember to check your skin products on EWG's Skin Deep site and ensure you only use products that score two or less in their database.

If you are in a job or play a sport where your face gets dirty, and you can't get rid of the dirt with just water, ensure you use a high-quality, slightly acidic shower gel or soap. You must also moisturise the skin afterwards, be it with aloe vera gel or another high-quality moisturiser.

---

[262] Eo et al., 2016
[263] Basmatker, et al., 2011

If wearing makeup, a good quality cleanser that removes the top layer of dead cells, oil, perspiration and pollution is necessary. If your skin is not cleansed properly, it will become dull and flaky, and the oil glands block up with dirt and cellular waste, causing breakouts and congestion.

To cleanse, gently press a warm, soft cloth against your face to soften and prepare the skin for cleansing. Shake the product well before use. Massage one or two pumps of cleanser into your face and neck, and remove with a damp cloth and plenty of water.

Purifying Face Masks

A purifying face mask can be used to draw toxins from the skin. These can be especially useful when initially starting out on your journey to great skin. Ingredients like charcoal and bentonite clay are often used to help draw toxins from the top layers of skin. These can be used after washing (with just water) and applying whilst the face (chest and back if affected) is still wet. Leave on for 15-20 minutes, then wash off with clean, warm water. Moisturise afterwards with aloe vera gel or another high-quality moisturiser.

Face masks should initially be used twice per week and reduced to once per week as the skin improves. However, be aware that they can, in the short-term, increase breakouts, but it is usually only temporary and leads to long-term benefits, so don't let a short-term response hold you back in the long run.

Good quality soaps, shower gels and face masks can be found in the resources section of the website at https://eliminateadultacne.com /resources.

Chapter summary/Key takeaways

- Skin cleansers work by removing dead skin cells, cleansing the pores, stimulating hormone- and oil-producing glands in the skin, improving circulation, assisting with the removal of stored toxins—including metabolic waste, heavy metals, excess minerals and environmental contaminants—and restoring optimal pH levels of the skin.

- Begin doing a daily skin brush.

- Alternate between the skin rub and vinegar baths.

- Your daily skin routine really is the cherry on top of the cake for helping you achieve clear skin for the rest of your life.

- Washing your face and other affected areas with plain, non-chlorinated water can be beneficial for maintaining the correct pH of the skin.

- For those who wear makeup or those needing to wash dirt, paint, and the like from their skin, it is important to use high-quality products, including a cleanser and moisturiser.

- Taking care of your skin on the outside, on top of all the other protocols taking care of it from the inside, will help ensure you have great skin for your next big event.

In the next chapter, in Part III, I show you how to put all of this information together to put it all into practice in an easy-to-follow manner.

SUCCESS STORY 7

Meet Simon.

Simon suffered from acne as a teenager and at the age of 21, began taking the antibiotic erythromycin. The erythromycin didn't work, and as a last resort, he took Accutane for four to five months. Whilst Simon had some good days on Accutane, he still had breakouts.

Simon was constantly anxious whenever the inevitable would happen and his skin would break out. From the age of 23-25, Simon went back on erythromycin, and again, the results were disappointing.

Simon came to see me at the age of 31 and immediately changed his diet, especially reducing foods that would spike his blood sugar. He introduced some essential supplements, started drinking more water, and reduced his alcohol intake to almost zero.

At the same time Simon started working with me, his doctor prescribed antibiotics for what he thought was Lyme disease, which was later diagnosed as a fungal rash.

Following the antibiotics, Simon started Saccharomyces boulardii to help rebalance his gut microbiome.

A couple of months in, Simon reported that his skin was as good as it had been in a long time. He has now experienced the longest spell without breakouts since he was a teenager.

Simon is no longer anxious about breakouts because he knows he's in control of how his skin looks with his lifestyle choices, which is very liberating for him.

It is amazing how simple the solution can be for some people. Simply reducing high glycaemic foods and lowering insulin levels was all Simon needed to do.

PART III

PUTTING IT ALL TOGETHER

PUTTING IT ALL TOGETHER

'Without knowledge action is useless and knowledge without action is futile.'

Abu Bakr

In this section, I give an overview of what to do every step of the way. I won't be going into detailing the 'how to' (that was covered in Section II), but I will give you an idea of when to do which step, in what order, for how long you need to do it, the fastest you are likely to complete it (in brackets) and how often you should repeat it.

Everyone goes at their own pace, but I will give you an idea of when to introduce each section at the earliest possible time so you can achieve clear skin consistently as soon as possible. However, I am a realist, and I understand that we all have different challenges in life, and therefore, you may have to take things a little slower, and that is 100% fine. Just be sure not to procrastinate before beginning your next task because you feel it is a little out of your comfort zone.

I often tell my clients, 'Nothing great has ever been achieved by staying in your comfort zone.' Staying in your comfort zone normally means you're not pushing or challenging yourself, and you're unlikely to achieve anything meaningful by staying in your comfort zone.

I'm sure that you are willing to go outside your comfort zone to achieve clear skin right now—if you ever feel like procrastinating, remember my phrase (above) and push yourself to do whatever it is that might seem a little uncomfortable at the time. You may also need to return to Step 1 to re-focus your mindset.

Believe me—the end result will be worth it.

In the tables for each chapter below, you will see tick boxes: one to tick when you start a specific task and another to tick once you've completed it. There is also a column to give you an idea of how long the task should take and how frequently you should do or repeat the task, and for how long.

You might find that just going through Steps 1 and 2 carefully and meticulously is all you need to achieve clear skin. You might find your skin clears quickly, and as long as you keep doing the right things, chances are your skin will stay clear going forwards. Going back to your old lifestyle is almost guaranteed to see the return of those dreaded breakouts.

If your skin does clear up quickly, it is up to you to decide whether to continue with the other steps. If achieving optimal health is important to you, then it would be a great idea to complete the remaining steps.

It may, however, be that you need to continue through one or more of the other steps to achieve everyday clear skin. My experience has shown me that some people's skin clears up in a few weeks, some a few months, and some might take 12-18 months.

Don't let that deter you; waking up each day without the anxiety of what might have appeared on your face overnight is worth the time and effort, not to mention all the other health benefits and the improvement of your confidence and self-esteem.

Please don't let the amount of lifestyle changes scare or deter you. Instead, be motivated by the fact that this might just be the most comprehensive plan you will ever find outside of receiving one-to-one coaching with a professional with a proven track record like myself.

If you are struggling to implement any of the protocols in his book and feel you could do with more help, take a look at my Eliminate Adult Acne Coaching Programme.

Details can be found at
https://skinwebinar.com.

Step 1–Setting Your Mindset for Success (Allow one Week):

Step 1 starts with setting your mindset for success. If you set aside one hour per day for the first five to seven days, you will set up the right mindset so it is in place for you to carry out all the necessary steps to achieve great skin every day.

It is important that you complete each of the steps in the order listed below (don't forget to revert back to Chapter 3 for the fine details of how to perform each task):

Chapter Three: Setting Your Mindset for Success	Started	Duration / Frequency	Completed
1. Set your goals. Write them down and have them printed out or on a mobile device where you will see them every day.	☐	<1 hour/ Yearly	☐
2. From your goals, create a positive affirmation statement.	☐	<1 hour/at least yearly	☐
3. Begin by repeating your positive affirmation statement daily. Feel as if you have already achieved your goal.	☐	Indefinitely/ multiple times daily	☐

4. Set your core values for each of the four doctors. Write them down and have them printed out or on a mobile device where you will see them every day. These are the rules you will live by to be successful.	☐	1-3 hours/ read daily, indefinitely	☐
5. Identify potential stumbling blocks to success. Write them down.	☐	< 1 hour	☐
6. List all solutions for over-coming your stumbling blocks before they happen. Write them down. Use this list to prepare ahead of challenging times, eliminating your excuse to fail.	☐	<1 hour	☐

If you feel as if things are taking too long, or you're not seeing results quickly enough, or you are losing motivation to stay on the programme, come back and repeat these exercises. It takes longer to reverse the damage for some than others. Stay focused and continue going through the processes. You can do this!

Step 2 - The Acne Elimination Diet (~ 3 Weeks):
Step 2 involves implementing all factors making up the Acne Elimination Diet. This stage usually takes between five to nine weeks to fully complete. You can begin incorporating the action points in Step 3 if you feel you have the capacity to do so, but don't stress yourself if you need to focus purely on Step 2.

Remember that each step builds upon the previous one, so keep on applying the principles of Step 1 (Chapter 3).

Chapter Four: The Acne Elimination Diet	Started	Duration / Frequency	Completed
1. Take the Metabolic Typing® Questionnaire – see https://eliminateadultacne.com /resources	☐	1-4 hours/ every 6 months	☐
2. Receive the results, including the Diet Plan. Cross off any foods from your plan known to cause acne.	☐	24 hours/ <1 hour	☐
3. Prepare a Four-Day Diet Plan (using the template provided).	☐	<1 hour/ quarterly	☐
4. Use the Four-Day Diet Plan to make your first grocery shopping list.	☐	<1 hour/ Repeat quarterly	☐
5. Complete your first Metabolic Typing® grocery shop. Buy as much food from organic sources as possible (plus wild, not farmed, fish organic or not).	☐	<1 hour/ every 4-7 days	☐
6. Start eating for your Metabolic Type® and eliminate any food known to cause acne.	☐	Indefinitely	☐

7. Begin the fine-tuning process by using the Diet Check Record Sheets (available at https://eliminateadultacne.com/resources).	☐	1-2 minutes/ 3 x per day	☐
8. Adjust your macronutrient ratios whenever you experience a poor response from a meal. Over time, this will help you 'dial in' to what your body needs.	☐	Until 'dialled in'	☐
9. Prepare to eat in a relaxed place, hydrate fully and chew your food until liquidised.	☐	30 minutes /2-3 x per day	☐
10. Introduce essential supplements one at a time. Wait at least three days before introducing the next supplement. Use only high-quality supplements.	☐	Every 3 days until maximised	☐
11. Test for food sensitivities (blood test or pulse test)	☐	3-4 weeks/ annually	☐
12. Begin replacing the foods you are sensitive to.	☐	Until complete	☐
13. Calculate your minimum requirement for water intake per day.	☐	< 2 mins/ daily/ indefinitely	☐

14. Choose/buy a high-quality source of water (RO-filtered or mineral water).	☐	Daily/ indefinitely	☐
15. Slowly increase your water intake by 0.25 litres per day (if required) each week until you hit your target.	☐	Daily until hitting target and maintain	☐
16. Slowly reduce/replace dehydrating beverages such as alcohol, caffeine, sodas, and fruit juices.	☐	A few days to a few weeks	☐

Step 3—Stress, Sleep & Rest (1-2 Weeks):

Most of the steps in this section can be introduced whilst completing Step 2 (The Acne Elimination Diet). As they don't take up extra time, it is more a case of rearranging your time. If you have mastered eating and hydrating correctly, you can also continue to work on Step 3 whilst working on Step 4 (Balancing the Gut-Skin Axis). However, you should NOT start Step 4 before mastering Step 2. Hopefully, that is clear.

Don't forget that you must still continue working on Steps 1 and 2.

Chapter Five: Stress, Sleep & Rest	Started	Duration / Frequency	Completed
1. Introduce a stress-reducing technique such as meditation, art therapy, sound therapy, massage, aromatherapy, cold and heat therapies, yoga, tai chi or qi gong.	☐	10-60 minutes per day/daily/ indefinitely	☐

	Started	Duration / Frequency	Completed
2. Begin going to bed 15 minutes earlier each week (until 10 pm becomes your normal bedtime).	☐	Daily until reached target	☐
3. Avoid all unnatural light one hour before bed.	☐	Every day/ indefinitely	☐
4. Remove all electrical devices from your bedroom.	☐	<1 hour/ indefinitely	☐
5. Ensure your bedroom is pitch-dark at night. Use blackout curtains and an eye mask if needed.	☐	Daily/ indefinitely	☐
6. Devise a pre-bed relax-ation/wind-down routine to help you sleep.	☐	30 minutes daily / indefinitely	☐
7. Turn off your wifi at night	☐	Daily/ indefinitely	☐
8. Use an earthing/grounding sheet to sleep on.	☐	Daily/ indefinitely	☐

Step 4—Balancing the Gut-Skin Axis (~18-20 Weeks):

Start this step only once you have mastered the Acne Elimination Diet. Don't forget that you must still work on Steps 1, 2 and 3.

To save time, order items you need in one go, which may also save money on postage.

Chapter Six: Balancing the Gut-Skin Axis	Started	Duration / Frequency	Completed
1. Introduce high-quality probiotic, prebiotic and/or fermented foods.	☐	Indefinitely	☐

2. Decide whether to have a stool test to assess your gut microbiome. If yes, find a functional medicine practitioner, naturopath or nutritionist to run the test for you.	☐	Results usually take 3-4 weeks	☐
3. To improve gut health and reduce gut permeability, introduce two or three of the following to your supplements protocol: zinc, glutamine, collagen peptides, deglycyrrhizinated liquorice (DGL), curcumin and/or omega-3 fatty acids.	☐	Use daily for at least 6 months	☐
4. Support your digestion with HCl (unless you have H Pylori), apple cider vinegar or Swedish bitters and possibly bile acids (if you don't have a gallbladder or you have an oily film around your stools).	☐	Use daily for at least 6 months	☐
5. Purchase the items to complete a heavy metal detox.	☐	Allow one week for delivery	☐
6. Complete the heavy metal detox, as instructed, for 90 days.	☐	<5 mins per day/90 days	☐

	Started	Duration / Frequency	Completed
7. Order supplements for the Body Ecology Cleanse	☐	~10 minutes	☐
8. Complete the Body Ecology Cleanse	☐	10-14 weeks	☐
9. Order supplements for the Intestinal Cleanse	☐	~10 minutes	☐
10. Complete the Intestinal Cleanse	☐	4-8 weeks/ Annually	☐

Step 5—The Outside-In Detox (~4-12 Weeks):

I suggest starting this after completing Step 4. However, there is no reason why you can't start these tasks beforehand. The reason I suggest starting after Step 4, is so you don't become overwhelmed with too many things to do or focus on.

Order the items you need in one go to save time.

Continue working on Steps 1, 2, 3 and 4.

Chapter Seven: The Outside-In Detox	Started	Duration / Frequency	Completed
1. Take steps to avoid (or give up) cigarette smoke and vapes.	☐	Varies with circumstances	☐
2. Plan to—and spend time in—nature (park, beach, forest, etc.) every day. Make this one of your important values.	☐	30 minutes daily	☐
3. If possible, use an air purifier in your home and work, or purchase air cleaner plants.	☐	Daily/ indefinitely	☐

4. If you have any metal fillings or root canal-filled teeth, see a biological or holistic dentist trained in the safe removal of metal fillings. This needs to be followed with a Heavy Metal Cleanse.	☐	Appointments vary on how many teeth require work. Replacing a root canal usually requires 2 treatments, 6 months apart.	☐
5. Check ALL of your personal care products in the www.ewg.org/skindeep database.	☐	30 minutes-1 hour	☐
6. Note which, if any, of your cookware items are made with non-stick coatings (Teflon), plastic, aluminium, copper or cast iron. Investigate alternatives for replacement.	☐	~10-minutes	☐
7. Plan and budget when you will replace each item.	☐	10-20 minutes	☐
8. Look into which of your household cleaning products need replacing.	☐	10-20 minutes	☐
9. Purchase less toxic cleaning products as you run out of the existing supply. Alternatively, throw away all of your toxic products and replace them immediately.	☐	10-20 minutes / indefinitely	☐

10. Throw away ALL toxic (plug-in) air fresheners immediately.	☐	<10 minutes	☐
11. Replace toxic air fresheners with pollutant-removing house plants and/or diffuse organic essential oils.		1-2 hours	
12. Use a dehumidifier if you live in a humid home, and consider professional advice if you have mould in your home.	☐	Use daily during waking hours, especially colder and wetter months	☐
13. Avoid buying cars less than three years old. Have your car cleaned inside and out regularly with biodegradable cleaning products and a cyclone vacuum cleaner.	☐	Cleaning: 1hour/ week	☐
14. If you use prescription medication, speak to your medical doctor about potentially reducing your dosage.	☐	Allow 1 hour for appointment. May require more than one appointment	☐

15. If you use recreational drugs, slowly reduce your intake to none and seek professional help if you are unable to do so without help.	☐	May take a few weeks to a few months	☐
16. Hire or purchase an EMF meter and analyse your home, workspace and car for electromagnetic radiation.	☐	Allow a week for delivery	☐
17. Minimise the harm by putting the EMR-reducing practical tips into place and purchasing EMR-protecting equipment where required.	☐	May take a few weeks to put into place/ indefinitely	☐
18. Begin a daily meditation practise (seated or moving) to reduce mental stress (if you haven't already).	☐	10-60 minutes daily	☐
19. Write a list of things you enjoy doing and a list of the things you dislike doing.	☐	< 1 hour/ quarterly	☐
20. Set aside time each week to plan how you will do more things you enjoy doing and fewer things you dislike doing…and then do it!	☐	At least 1 hour per week/ indefinitely	☐

Step 6 - The Inside-Out Detox (~12 Weeks):

I suggest starting this after completing Step 5. Whilst you can start Step 6 earlier, you will achieve better results once you have minimised the amount of toxins consumed every day via your skin, breath, and mouth. Starting Step 6 after Step 5 also prevents being overwhelmed by trying to do too many things at once.

To save time, order the equipment you need and purchase it together. This will also save money on postage.

Continue working on Steps 1, 2, 3, 4 and 5.

Chapter Eight: The Inside-Out Detox	Started	Duration / Frequency	Completed
1. Purchase or build your own infrared sauna or find a facility near you that has one.	☐	Allow yourself 3-4 weeks	☐
2. Take an infrared sauna daily. Follow the instructions in Chapter 8 carefully. Get permission from your doctor first.	☐	Use daily for at least 6 months	☐
3. Purchase the items required to complete the coffee enemas.	☐	Allow one week for delivery	☐
4. Begin coffee enemas following the instructions in Chapter 8. Get permission from your doctor first.	☐	Allow 1 hour per day/ every other day for 4 months	☐
5. Purchase the items required to complete a Colon Cleanse.	☐	Allow one week for delivery	☐

6. Complete a Colon Cleanse.	☐	7-day prep & 3-day cleanse/ annually	☐
7. Purchase the items to complete Castor Oil Packs.	☐	Allow one week for delivery	☐
8. Complete daily Castor Packs for 5-days leading up to a Liver/Gallbladder Cleanse and whenever you desire.	☐	1-1.5 hours daily/5 days+	☐
9. Purchase the items to complete Liver/Gallbladder Cleanses.	☐	Allow one week for delivery	☐
10. Complete a Liver/ Gallbladder Cleanse monthly (at the beginning).	☐	6 days/ monthly to start and then twice per year	☐
11. Purchase the items to complete to complete Cell Cleanses.	☐	Allow one week for delivery	☐
12. Complete a Cell Cleanse.	☐	2 days/1-2 per year	☐
13. Purchase the items to complete to complete Skin Cleanses.	☐	Allow one week for delivery	☐
14. Complete daily Skin Cleanses as instructed in Chapter 8.	☐	30-minutes /1-2 per week	☐

If you are struggling to implement any of the protocols in his book and feel you could do with more help, I do have a coaching programme—Eliminate Adult Acne—the details of which can be found at

https://skinwebinar.com.

Step 7 - The Skin Cleansing Ritual (~1-2 Weeks):

You can start Step 7 at any time. The reason it is last in this book is because it will have the smallest effect when it comes to reducing your acne. It is like the cherry on top of the cake, so to speak. Continue working on Steps 1, 2, 3, 4, 5 and 6.

Chapter Nine: The Skin Cleansing Ritual	Started	Duration / Frequency	Completed
1. Check out your personal care products (if you haven't already) at www.ewg.org/skindeep to see how safe or toxic they are.	☐	30 minutes-1 hour	☐
2. Research whole-house water filtration systems.	☐	1-2 hours	☐
3. Purchase a whole house filtration system for bathing water.	☐	Use daily/ indefinitely	☐
4. Wash only your 'pits' and 'bits' with a high-quality soap or shower gel. Wash the rest of your body, including your face, with clean water only.	☐	Daily/ indefinitely	☐

5. Use a good moisturiser after washing, such as organic aloe vera gel.	☐	A few seconds daily/ indefinitely	☐
6. If you feel like your skin is toxic, use a high-quality purifying face mask.	☐	20 minutes/ 1-2 per week	☐

Regular Tasks

Below is an overview of the tasks required to achieve great skin on a daily, weekly, quarterly, and annual basis. It may seem overwhelming at first glance, but by making slow changes over time, these tasks will become a part of your everyday life. It will soon become the way you live your life as it did for me, and it will be a life in which you do not have the stress, anxiety or worry over how your skin will look.

These tasks will help you have clear skin every day and regain your confidence and self-esteem.

Tasks	Daily	Weekly	Quarterly	Annually
Positive Affirmation Statements	Yes			
Set Your Core Values				Yes
Take Metabolic Typing® Test				Twice
Prepare 4-Day Diet Plan			Yes	
Eat right for your Metabolic Type®	Yes			
Test for food sensitivities				Yes
Drink optimal amounts of good-quality water	Yes			
Stress-Reducing Technique	Yes			

Pre-bed wind-down routine	Yes			
Sleep on a grounding sheet	Yes			
Take high-quality MT® specific supplements	2-3 times			
Run a GI Stool Test				Annually (+follow up if needed)
Take Gut healing supplements	Yes			
Heavy Metal Detox	Yes (1st 90 days)			
Complete a Body Ecology Cleanse				If needed
Complete an Intestinal Cleanse				Yes
Spend time in nature	Yes			
Use high-quality personal care products	Yes			
Use only toxic-free cookware	2-3 times			
Use safe home cleaning products	Yes			
Use dehumidifier (if required)	Yes			
Use EMF protection devices	Yes			
Do things you enjoy/love to do	Yes			

Infrared sauna		2-5 times		
Coffee enemas	Yes (ini-tially)			
Colon Cleanse			Yes	
Liver/Gallbladder Cleanse			Yes	
Cell Cleanse				Twice
Skin Cleanse			Yes	
Wash face with 'clean' water only	1-2 times			
Only wash 'pits' & 'bits' with soap	1-2 times			
Purifying face mask		1-2 times		

CONCLUSION

A s someone who has walked the acne path, the steps required to achieve great skin every day might seem like a lot of work, but it really is worth it. Once you have made the initial lifestyle changes, they will become a part of your everyday life. Not only will your skin improve, but many aspects of your health will improve along with it.

By ensuring you eat right for your Metabolic Type®, avoiding food you are sensitive to, and food known to cause acne, you will travel far down the path toward clear skin. Balancing your microbiome, minimising exposure to environmental toxins and detoxing from the inside out will take the toxic load off of your detoxification systems, simply giving your skin room to breathe without having to purge the toxins for you.

I can honestly say that I never think about how my skin is going to be these days. That stress, anxiety and worry about how my skin will look when I wake up simply aren't there anymore, and it hasn't been for a long time. I sometimes forget how bad it was and how badly acne affected my life. I really want you to feel the same way. It is my hope that, following the guidance in this book, you will look back in the years to come, having forgotten how badly your acne once affected you.

Here's to clear skin and success in the future as you lead a more confident, fun-filled, healthy, productive and fulfilling life!

ABOUT THE AUTHOR

After suffering from acne for 18 years, the year 2000 was a turning point for Leigh as he found the teachers and knowledge he needed to cure his acne. Since then, he has been passionate about learning more and turning the learning into wisdom through experience in what is now almost 30 years of working with clients.

Leigh always sought the 'best of the best' to learn from and is as passionate about his work and gaining knowledge now as he was in 1996 when his career in health, wellness and performance started.

Leigh has studied many different disciplines, including holistic dermatology, nutrition, functional medicine, corrective exercise, strength and conditioning, tennis conditioning, energy medicine, BioGeometry and manual therapy, to name a few. This has given him the ability to provide a truly holistic approach when helping his clients over the years, which they have often times found effective when other approaches haven't helped.

Leigh has formally studied with some of the world's greatest minds, such as Paul Chek, Bill Wolcott, Dr John Veltheim (RIP), Dr Michael Leahy, and Dr Dietrich Klinghardt.

As well as being passionate about helping clients, he has been a member of the faculty of the world-renowned CHEK Institute, working alongside CHEK Institute founder Paul Chek since 2010, teaching and presenting in Europe, the USA and Australia.

Leigh has also authored *Anatomy of Strength for Fitness Training in Speed for Sport, Anatomy of Yoga for Posture & Health, Anatomy of*

Sports Injuries for Training & Rehabilitation and *The Tennis Biomechanics Manual*. Leigh also provides online coaching and education programmes, such as HEAL THEM Education for health professionals (www.healthemeducation.com) and the Eliminate Adult Acne online coaching programme for acne sufferers (www.eliminateadultacne.com).

In 2022, Leigh started *The Radical Health Rebel Podcast* (www.radicalhealthrebel.com), which includes weekly discussions and interviews on all things health and wellness, with a focus on skin health, gut health, chronic pain and more, for health enthusiasts and those seeking to overcome specific health challenges.

Outside of work, Leigh has a passion for music, especially dance music and lifting weights at the gym. He loves to get out on the tennis court at least once a week, as well as going into nature for long walks near his home in Hertfordshire, England.

Leigh's Eliminate Adult Acne Coaching Programme details can be found at https://skinwebinar.com.

Leigh can also be found at:

https://www.youtube.com/@radicalhealthrebelpodcast
https://www.instagram.com/radicalhealthrebel/
https://www.facebook.com/radicalhealthrebel/
https://twitter.com/leighbrandon

APPENDICES

SLOW OXIDISER DIET PLAN

Eating Guidelines for Axe Adult Acne

4/15/2013

Food Colors

Green = ideal (eat ideal foods at every meal)
Black = Neutral (ok. but emphasize "ideal" foods)
Italics = Caution (eat rarely or only for variety)
Red = Avoid (don't eat these foods)

Meats

Pork (ham, chops); *Beef*; Lamb; *Pork (bacon)*; Buffalo; *Elk*; Heart (beef); Kidney (beef); Liver (beef); Rabbit; Venison

Poultry

Chicken (dark meat); Chicken (white meat); Cornish Hen; Turkey (dark meat); Turkey (white meat); *Duck*; Goose; *Pheasant*; *Quail*

Seafood

Bass (freshwater)	Snapper	Shrimp
Bass (sea)	*Swordfish*	*Squid*
Catfish	Tuna	*Trout*
Cod	Whitefish	Anchovy
Grouper	*Abalone*	Caviar
Halibut	*Clams*	Herring
Mahi-mahi	*Crab*	Mackerel
Perch	*Crayfish*	Mussels
Pompano	*Lobster*	Sardines
Rockfish	*Octopus*	Scallop
Roughy	*Oysters*	
Shark	*Salmon*	

Legumes

Garbanzo Beans	**Lima Beans**
Navy Beans	**Mung Beans**
Pinto Beans	**Red Beans**
White Beans	Black-eyed-Peas
Azuki) Beans	Soy-Beans
Black Beans	Tofu
Fava Beans	
Great Northern Beans	
Green Beans	
Lentils	

Beverages

Oat Milk	Liquor
Tea (green)	Rice-Milk
Tea (herbal)	Soft-Drinks-(colas)
Vegetable Juices	Soy-Milk
Water (pure, bottled)	Water (carbonated)
Almond Milk	Water (tap)
Coffee (decaf)	Wine (red)
Water (distilled)	Wine (white)
Coffee (caffeinated)	
Tea (black)	
Beer	
Fruit Juices	

Dairy and Eggs

Eggs, Chicken (whites)	Ice-Cream
Eggs, Chicken (yolks)	Milk-(2%)
Eggs, Duck (whole)	Milk-(skim)
Blue-Cheese	Milk-(whole)
Buttermilk	Monterey-Jack
Brie	Mozzarella
Camembert	Muenster
Cheddar	Neufchatel
Colby	Parmesan
Cottage-Cheese	Provolone
Cottage-Cheese-(lite)	Ricotta
Cream-(half-and-half)	Romano
Cream-Cheese	Roquefort
Edam	Sorbet
Feta	Sour-Cream
Goat-Cheese	Swiss
Goat-Milk	Whey
Gouda	Yogurt
Gruyere	

Nuts and Seeds

Almonds	*Brazil Nuts*
Cashews	*Filberts*
Chestnuts	Macadamia Nuts
Hickory Nuts	Peanuts
Pecans	
Pine Nuts	
Pistachios	
Poppy Seeds	
Pumpkin Seeds	
Sesame Seeds	
Sunflower Seeds	
Walnuts	

Grains

Amaranth	**Barley**
Kamut	**Buckwheat**
Quinoa	**Millet**
Spelt	**Oats**
Triticale	Rice (basmati)
	Rice (brown)
	Rice (plain, white)
	Rye
	Wheat
	Wild Rice

Greens

Arugula; Beet Greens; Cilantro; Collard Greens; Dandelion Greens; Endive; Kale; Lettuce (bibb); Lettuce (iceberg); Lettuce (loose-leaf); Lettuce (romaine); Mustard Greens; Radicchio; Spinach; Sprouts (alfalfa); Sprouts (bean); Swiss Chard; Turnip Greens; Watercress

Vegetables

Asparagus	**Water Chestnuts**	Squash (summer)
Bamboo Shoots	**Zucchini**	Squash (winter)
Bok Choy	Artichoke	Sweet-Potato-(yam)
Broccoli	Avocado	Tomatoes
Brussels Sprout	Cauliflower	
Cabbage	Celery	
Carrots	Fennel	
Cucumber	Garlic	
Daikon	Ginger Root	
Eggplant	Jerusalem Artichoke	
Jicama	Mushroom (all varieties)	
Kohlrabi	Okra	
Leek	Olive (all varieties)	
Parsnip	Onions	
Pepper (bell, all colors)	Rutabaga	
Pepper (hot, all colors)	Turnip	
Pumpkin	Beets	
Radish	Corn	
Shallot	Potato (all varieties)	

Sea Vegetables

Dulse; Laver; Agar; Irish Moss (carrageenan); Kelp; Wakame

Fruits

Apples	Kiwifruit	
Apricots	Kumquat	
Blackberries	Lemons	
Blueberries	Limes	
Boysenberries	Oranges	
Casaba Melon	Prunes	
Cherries	Tangerines	
Coconut	Banana	
Cranberries	Cantaloupe	
Elderberries	Dates	
Gooseberries	Figs	
Grapefruit	Pineapple	
Grapes	Raisins	
Guava	Watermelon	
Honeydew Melon	Currants	

Oils and Fats

Borage Oil	*Sesame Oil*
Coconut Oil	*Sunflower Oil*
Evening Primrose Oil	*Wheat Germ Oil*
Fish Oils	Canola Oil
Flaxseed Oil	Corn Oil
Olive Oil	Cottonseed-Oil
Palm Kernel Oil	Margarine
Almond Oil	
Black Currant Oil	
Butter (salted)	
Butter (unsalted)	
Ghee (clarified butter)	
Hemp Oil	
Peanut Oil	
Safflower Oil	

Herbs, Spices and Seasonings

Anise	Fennel Seed	Sage	Vanilla (extract)
Basil	Fenugreek	Salt (sea salt, unrefined)	Vinegar (balsamic)
Bay Leaf	Ginger	Savory	Vinegar (rice)
Caraway	Mace	Soy Sauce	Artificial-Sweeteners
Cardamom	Marjoram	Spearmint	Chocolate
Cayenne	Mustard	Tarragon	Honey
Chervil	Mustard Seed	Thyme	Ketchup
Chili Powder	Nutmeg	Turmeric	Salt (iodized)
Chive	Oregano	Wasabi	Salt (low-sodium)
Cinnamon	Paprika	Carob	Sugar (brown)
Cloves	Parsley	Garlic Powder	Sugar (white)
Coriander	Pepper (ground black)	Horseradish	Sugar (brown, unrefined)
Cumin	Peppermint	Vinegar (apple cider)	Vinegar (wine)
Curry Powder	Rosemary	*Mayonnaise*	
Dill Weed	Saffron	*Molasses*	

These Eating Guidelines may require modification as your health status changes. Schedule a follow-up with your practitioner.

FAST OXIDISER DIET PLAN

Eating Guidelines for Axe Adult Acne

Food Colors
Green = Ideal (eat ideal foods at every meal)
Black = Neutral (ok, but emphasize "ideal" foods)
Italics = Caution (eat rarely or only for variety)
Red = Avoid (don't eat these foods)

15/04/2013

Meats
Beef, Buffalo, Elk, Heart (beef), Kidney (beef), Lamb, Liver (beef), Pork (bacon), Pork (ham, chops), Rabbit, Venison

Poultry
Chicken (dark meat), Duck, Goose, Pheasant, Quail, Turkey (dark meat), **Chicken (white meat)**, **Cornish Hen**, **Turkey (white meat)**

Seafood
Abalone, Anchovy, Catfish, Caviar, Clams, Crab, Crayfish, Herring, Lobster, Mussels, Octopus, Oysters, Perch, Pompano, Salmon, Sardines, Scallop, Shark, Shrimp, Squid, Swordfish, Trout, Tuna, Whitefish, *Bass (freshwater)*, *Bass (sea)*, *Cod*, *Grouper*, *Halibut*, *Mahi-mahi*, *Rockfish*, *Roughy*, *Snapper*

Grains
Amaranth, Kamut, Quinoa, Spelt, Triticale, *Barley*, *Buckwheat*, *Millet*, *Oats*, *Rice (basmati)*, *Rice (brown)*, *Rice (plain, white)*, *Rye*, Wheat, *Wild Rice*

Beverages
Water (pure, bottled), **Almond Milk**, **Water (distilled)**, *Coffee (decaf)*, *Tea (black)*, *Tea (green)*, *Tea (herbal)*, *Vegetable Juices*, Beer, Coffee (caffeinated), Fruit-Juices, Oat-Milk, Rice-Milk, Soft Drinks (colas), Soy-Milk, Spirits, Water (carbonated), Water (tap), Wine (red), Wine (white)

Sea Vegetables
Agar, Dulse, Irish Moss (carrageenan), Kelp, Wakame, **Laver**

Dairy and Eggs
Eggs, Chicken (yolks), Eggs, Duck (whole), **Eggs, Chicken (whites)**, *Ice-Cream*, *Milk (semi-skimmed)*, *Milk (skimmed)*, *Milk (whole)*, Blue-Cheese, Brie, Buttermilk, Monterey-Jack, Camembert, Mozzarella, Cheddar, Muenster, Colby, Neufchatel, Cottage-Cheese, Parmesan, Cottage-Cheese (low fat), Provolone, Cream (bright), Ricotta, Cream-Cheese, Romano, Cream-Cheese, Roquefort, Edam, Sorbet, Feta, Sour-Cream, Goat-Cheese, Swiss, Goat-Milk, Whey, Gouda, Yogurt, Gruyere

Nuts and Seeds
Brazil Nuts, Filberts, Hickory Nuts, Macadamia Nuts, Peanuts, Pecans, Pumpkin Seeds, Walnuts, **Almonds**, **Pistachios**, **Sesame Seeds**, *Cashews*, *Chestnuts*, *Pine Nuts*, *Poppy Seeds*, *Sunflower Seeds*

Greens
Spinach, Watercress, *Lettuce (iceberg)*, *Lettuce (loose-leaf)*, *Lettuce (romaine)*, *Lettuce (round)*, Spring Greens, Turnip Greens, Coriander, Dandelion Greens, Kale, Radicchio, Rocket, Sprouts (alfalfa), Sprouts (bean), Chard, Beetroot-Greens, Endive, Mustard-Greens

Legumes
Azuki Beans, Black Beans, Broad Beans, Butter Beans, Great Northern Beans, Green Beans, Green Peas, Kidney Beans, Lentils, Mung Beans, Navy Beans, **Pink Beans**, **Pinto Beans**, **White Beans**, Black-eyed Peas, Soy-Beans, Tofu, Chickpeas

Vegetables
Artichoke, Asparagus, Avocado, Carrots, Cauliflower, Celery, Jerusalem Artichoke, Mushroom (all varieties), Olive (all varieties), **Okra**, **Turnip**, Aubergine, Bamboo Shoots, Bok Choy, Cabbage, Courgette, Cucumber, Daikon (asian radish), Fennel, *Ginger Root*, *Jicama*, *Kohlrabi*, *Radish*, *Swede*, *Water Chestnuts*, Beetroot, Broccoli, Brussels-Sprout, Butternut-Squash, Garlic, Leek, Onions, Parsnip, Pepper (bell, all colors), Pepper (hot, all colors), Potato (all varieties), Pumpkin, Shallot, Squash (summer), Sweet-Potato (yam), Sweetcorn, Tomatoes

Oils and Fats
Sesame Oil, Sunflower Oil, Wheat Germ Oil, Canola-Oil, Corn-Oil, Cottonseed-Oil, Margarine, *Borage Oil*, *Coconut Oil*, *Evening Primrose Oil*, *Fish Oils*, *Linseed Oil*, *Olive Oil*, *Palm Kernel Oil*, Almond Oil, Black Currant Oil, Butter (salted), Butter (unsalted), Ghee (clarified butter), Hemp Oil, Peanut Oil, Safflower Oil

Herbs, Spices and Seasonings
Anise, Basil, Bay Leaf, Caraway, Cardamom, Cayenne, Chervil, Chilli Powder, Chive, Cinnamon, Coriander, Cloves, Cumin, Curry Powder, Dill, Fennel Seed, Fenugreek, Ginger, Mace, Marjoram, Nutmeg, Oregano, Paprika, Pepper (ground black), Peppermint, Rosemary, Saffron, Sal (sea salt, unrefined), Sage, Savory, Soy Sauce, Spearmint, Tarragon, Thyme, Turmeric, **Vanilla (extract)**, Carob, Mayonnaise, Molasses, Vinegar (apple cider), Wasabi, Artificial-Sweeteners, Chocolate, Garlic-Powder, Honey, Horseradish, Ketchup, Mustard, Mustard-Seed, Parsley, Salt (iodized), Salt (low-sodium), Sugar (brown), Sugar (white), Sugar (brown, unrefined), Vinegar (balsamic), Vinegar (rice), Vinegar (wine)

Fruits
Apples, Coconut, Pears, *Apricots*, *Blackberries*, *Blueberries*, *Boysenberries*, *Cherries*, *Cranberries*, *Elderberries*, *Gooseberries*, *Guava*, *Kiwifruit*, *Kumquat*, *Loganberries*, Mango, Nectarines, Papaya, Peaches, Plums, Pomegranate, Raspberries, Rhubarb, Strawberries, Banana, Cantaloupe, Casaba Melon, Currants, Dates, Figs, Grapefruit, Grapes, Honeydew-Melon, Lemons, Limes, Oranges, Persimmon, Pineapple, Prunes, Raisins, Tangerines, Watermelon

These Eating Guidelines may require modification as your health status changes. Schedule a follow-up with your practitioner.

MIXED OXIDISER DIET PLAN

Eating Guidelines for Axe Adult Acne

15/04/2013

Food Colors

Green = Option #1 (eat either Option #1 or #2 at a meal, but not both)
Purple = Option #2 (eat either Option #1 or #2 at a meal, but not both)
Black = Neutral (eat freely with Option #1 or #2)
Italics = Caution (eat only rarely)
Red = Avoid (don't eat these foods)

Meats
Beef, Buffalo, Elk, Heart (beef), Kidney (beef), Lamb, Liver (beef), Pork (bacon), Rabbit, Venison, Pork (ham, chops)

Poultry
Chicken (dark meat), Duck, Goose, Pheasant, Quail, Turkey (dark meat), Chicken (white meat), Cornish Hen, Turkey (white meat)

Seafood
Abalone, Anchovy, Catfish, Caviar, Clams, Crab, Crayfish, Herring, Lobster, Mackerel, Mussels, Octopus, Oysters, Perch, Pompano, Salmon, Sardines, Scallop, Shark, Shrimp, Squid, Swordfish, Trout, Tuna, Whitefish, Bass (freshwater), Bass (sea), Cod, Grouper, Halibut, Mahi-mahi, Rockfish, Roughy, Snapper

Greens
Beetroot Greens, Chard, Coriander, Dandelion Greens, Endive, Kale, Mustard Greens, Radicchio, Rocket, Sprouts (alfalfa), Sprouts (bean), Lettuce (iceberg), Lettuce (loose-leaf), Lettuce (romaine), Lettuce (round), Spinach, Spring Greens, Turnip Greens, Watercress

Grains
Spelt, Triticale, Amaranth, Kamut, Quinoa, Barley, Buckwheat, Oats, Millet, Rice (basmati), Rice (brown), Rice (plain, white), Rye, Wheat, Wild Rice

Oils and Fats
Fish Oils, Linseed Oil, Borage Oil, Coconut Oil, Evening Primrose Oil, Olive Oil, Palm Kernel Oil, Almond Oil, Black Currant Oil, Butter (salted), Butter (unsalted), Ghee (clarified butter), Hemp Oil, Peanut Oil, Safflower Oil, Sesame Oil, Sunflower Oil, Wheat Germ Oil, Canola Oil, Corn Oil, Cottonseed Oil, Margarine

Dairy and Eggs
Eggs, Chicken (yolks), Eggs, Duck (whole), Eggs, Chicken (whites), Blue-Cheese, Brie, Buttermilk, Camembert, Cheddar, Colby, Cottage-Cheese, Cottage-Cheese (low-fat), Cream (single), Cream-Cheese, Edam, Feta, Goat-Cheese, Gouda, Gruyere, Ice-Cream, Milk (semi-skimmed), Milk (skimmed), Milk (whole), Monterey-Jack, Mozzarella, Muenster, Neufchatel, Parmesan, Provolone, Ricotta, Romano, Roquefort, Sorbet, Sour-Cream, Swiss, Whey, Yogurt

Nuts and Seeds
Almonds, Cashews, Chestnuts, Pine Nuts, Pistachios, Poppy Seeds, Sesame Seeds, Sunflower Seeds, Brazil Nuts, Filberts, Hickory Nuts, Macadamia Nuts, Peanuts, Pecans, Pumpkin Seeds, Walnuts

Fruits
Apricots, Cherries, Papaya, Persimmon, Apples, Blackberries, Blueberries, Boysenberries, Casaba Melon, Coconut, Cranberries, Elderberries, Gooseberries, Grapes, Guava, Honeydew Melon, Kiwifruit, Kumquat, Loganberries, Mango, Nectarines, Peaches, Pears, Plums, Pomegranate, Raspberries, Rhubarb, Strawberries, Currants, Grapefruit, Lemons, Limes, Oranges, Prunes, Tangerines, Banana, Cantaloupe, Dates, Figs, Pineapple, Raisins, Watermelon

Legumes
Chickpeas, Navy Beans, Pink Beans, Pinto Beans, White Beans, Azuki Beans, Black Beans, Broad Beans, Butter Beans, Great Northern Beans, Green Beans, Green Peas, Kidney Beans, Lentils, Mung Beans, Black-eyed-Peas, Soy-Beans, Tofu

Vegetables
Aubergine, Bamboo Shoots, Bok Choy, Broccoli, Brussels Sprout, Cabbage, Courgette, Cucumber, Daikon (asian radish), Fennel, Garlic, Ginger Root, Jicama, Kohlrabi, Leek, Onions, Parsnip, Pepper (bell, all colors), Pepper (hot, all colors), Pumpkin, Radish, Shallot, Swede, Water Chestnuts, Artichoke, Asparagus, Avocado, Carrots, Cauliflower, Celery, Jerusalem Artichoke, Mushroom (all varieties), Okra, Olive (all varieties), Turnip, Beetroot, Butternut-Squash, Potato (all varieties), Squash (summer), Sweet-Potato-(yam), Sweetcorn, Tomatoes

Herbs, Spices and Seasonings
Anise, Basil, Bay Leaf, Caraway, Cardamom, Carob, Cayenne, Chervil, Chilli Powder, Chive, Cinnamon, Cloves, Coriander, Cumin, Curry Powder, Dill, Fennel Seed, Fenugreek, Garlic Powder, Ginger, Horseradish, Mace, Marjoram, Mayonnaise, Molasses, Mustard, Mustard Seed, Nutmeg, Oregano, Paprika, Parsley, Pepper (ground black), Peppermint, Rosemary, Saffron, Sage, Salt (sea salt, unrefined), Savory, Soy Sauce, Spearmint, Tarragon, Thyme, Turmeric, Vanilla (extract), Vinegar (apple cider), Vinegar (balsamic), Vinegar (rice), Wasabi, Artificial-Sweeteners, Chocolate, Honey, Ketchup, Salt (iodised), Salt (low-sodium), Sugar (brown), Sugar (white), Sugar (brown-unrefined), Vinegar (wine)

Beverages
Almond Milk, Coffee (caffeinated), Coffee (decaf), Oat Milk, Tea (black), Tea (green), Tea (herbal), Vegetable Juices, Water (distilled), Water (pure, bottled), Beer, Fruit-Juices, Rice-Milk, Soft-Drinks-(colas), Soy-Milk, Spirits, Water-(carbonated), Water-(top), Wine-(red), Wine-(white)

Sea Vegetables
Dulse, Nori, Agar, Irish Moss(carrageenan), Kelp, Wakame

These Eating Guidelines may require modification as your health status changes. Schedule a follow-up with your practitioner

Eating Guidelines for Axe Adult Acne

APPENDIX 4

SYMPATHETIC DIET PLAN

Food Colors

Green = Ideal (eat ideal foods at every meal)
Black = Neutral (ok, but emphasize "ideal" foods)
Italics = Caution (eat rarely or only for variety)
Red = Avoid (don't eat these foods)

Meats

Pork (ham, chops)
Beef
Lamb
Pork (bacon)
Buffalo
Elk
Heart (beef)
Kidney (beef)
Liver (beef)
Rabbit
Venison

Poultry

Chicken (dark meat)
Chicken (white meat)
Cornish Hen
Turkey (dark meat)
Turkey (white meat)
Duck
Goose
Pheasant
Quail

Seafood

Bass (freshwater)
Bass (sea)
Catfish
Cod
Grouper
Halibut
Mahi-mahi
Perch
Pompano
Rockfish
Roughy
Shark
Snapper
Swordfish
Tuna
Whitefish
Clams
Crab
Crayfish
Lobster
Octopus
Oysters
Salmon
Shrimp
Squid
Trout
Anchovy
Caviar
Herring
Mackerel
Mussels
Sardines
Scallop

Legumes

Garbanzo Beans
Navy Beans
Pinto Beans
White Beans
Azuki Beans
Black Beans
Fava Beans
Great Northern Beans
Green Beans
Green Peas
Lentils
Lima Beans
Mung Beans
Red Beans
Black-eyed Peas
Soy Beans
Tofu

Beverages

Oat Milk
Tea (green)
Tea (herbal)
Vegetable Juices
Water (pure, bottled)
Almond Milk
Coffee (decaf)
Water (distilled)
Coffee (caffinated)
Tea (black)
Beer
Fruit Juices
Liquor
Rice Milk
Soft Drinks (colas)
Soy Milk
Water (carbonated)
Water (tap)
Wine (red)
Wine (white)

Dairy and Eggs

Eggs, Chicken (white)
Eggs, Chicken (yolks)
Eggs, Duck (whole)
Blue Cheese
Brie
Buttermilk
Camembert
Cheddar
Colby
Cottage Cheese
Cottage Cheese (lite)
Cream (half-and-half)
Cream Cheese
Edam
Feta
Goat Cheese
Goat Milk
Gouda
Gruyere
Ice Cream
Milk (2%)
Milk (skim)
Milk (whole)
Monterey-Jack
Mozzarella
Muenster
Neufchatel
Parmesan
Provolone
Ricotta
Romano
Roquefort
Sorbet
Sour Cream
Swiss
Whey
Yogurt

Nuts and Seeds

Almonds
Cashews
Chestnuts
Hickory Nuts
Pecans
Pine Nuts
Pistachios
Poppy Seeds
Pumpkin Seeds
Sesame Seeds
Sunflower Seeds
Walnuts
Brazil Nuts
Filberts
Macadamia Nuts
Peanuts

Grains

Amaranth
Kamut
Quinoa
Spelt
Triticale
Barley
Buckwheat
Millet
Oats
Rice (basmati)
Rice (brown)
Rice (plain, white)
Rye
Wheat
Wild-Rice

Vegetables

Water Chestnuts
Zucchini
Artichoke
Avocado
Cauliflower
Celery
Fennel
Garlic
Ginger Root
Jerusalem Artichoke
Mushroom (all varieties)
Olive (all varieties)
Onions
Rutabaga
Turnip
Beets
Potato (all varieties)
Squash (summer)
Squash (winter)
Sweet Potato (yam)
Tomatoes

Sea Vegetables

Dulse
Laver
Irish Moss (carrageenan)
Agar
Kelp
Wakame

Fruits

Apples
Apricots
Blackberries
Blueberries
Boysenberries
Casaba Melon
Cherries
Coconut
Cranberries
Elderberries
Gooseberries
Grapefruit
Grapes
Guava
Honeydew Melon
Kiwifruit
Kumquat
Loganberries
Mango
Nectarines
Papaya
Peaches
Pears
Persimmon
Plums
Pomegranate
Raspberries
Rhubarb
Strawberries
Currants
Lemons
Limes
Oranges
Prunes
Tangerines
Banana
Cantaloupe
Dates
Figs
Pineapple
Raisins
Watermelon

Greens

Arugula
Beet Greens
Cilantro
Collard Greens
Dandelion Greens
Endive
Kale
Lettuce (bibb)
Lettuce (iceberg)
Lettuce (loose-leaf)
Lettuce (romaine)
Mustard Greens
Radicchio
Spinach
Sprouts (alfalfa)
Sprouts (bean)
Swiss Chard
Turnip Greens
Watercress
Shrimp
Squid
Trout
Anchovy
Caviar
Herring
Mackerel
Mussels
Sardines
Scallop

Vegetables

Asparagus
Bamboo Shoots
Bok Choy
Broccoli
Brussels Sprout
Cabbage
Carrots
Cucumber
Daikon
Eggplant
Jicama
Kohlrabi
Leek
Parsnip
Pepper (bell, all colors)
Pepper (hot, all colors)
Pumpkin
Radish
Shallot

Oils and Fats

Borage Oil
Coconut Oil
Evening Primrose Oil
Fish Oils
Flaxseed Oil
Olive Oil
Palm Kernel Oil
Almond Oil
Black Currant Oil
Butter (salted)
Butter (unsalted)
Ghee (clarified butter)
Hemp Oil
Peanut Oil
Safflower Oil
Sesame Oil
Sunflower Oil
Wheat Germ Oil
Corn Oil
Cottonseed Oil
Margarine

Herbs, Spices and Seasonings

Fennel Seed
Fenugreek
Ginger
Mace
Marjoram
Mustard
Mustard Seed
Nutmeg
Oregano
Paprika
Parsley
Pepper (ground black)
Peppermint
Rosemary
Saffron
Anise
Basil
Bay Leaf
Caraway
Cardamom
Cayenne
Chervil
Chili Powder
Chive
Cinnamon
Cloves
Coriander
Cumin
Curry Powder
Dill Weed
Sage
Salt (sea salt, unrefined)
Savory
Soy Sauce
Spearmint
Tarragon
Thyme
Turmeric
Wasabi
Carob
Garlic Powder
Horseradish
Vinegar (apple cider)
Mayonnaise
Molasses
Vanilla (extract)
Vinegar (balsamic)
Vinegar (rice)
Artificial Sweeteners
Chocolate
Honey
Ketchup
Salt (iodized)
Salt (low-sodium)
Sugar (brown)
Sugar (white)
Sugar (brown, unrefined)
Vinegar (wine)

These Eating Guidelines may require modification as your health status changes. Schedule a follow-up with your practitioner.

PARASYMPATHETIC DIET PLAN

15/04/2013

Eating Guidelines for Axe Adult Acne

Food Colors

Green = Ideal (eat ideal foods at every meal)
Black = Neutral (ok, but emphasize "ideal" foods)
Italics = Caution (eat rarely or only for variety)
Red = Avoid (don't eat these foods)

Meats
Beef, Buffalo, Elk, Heart (beef), Kidney (beef), Lamb, Liver (beef), Pork (bacon), Pork (ham, chops), Rabbit, Venison

Poultry
Chicken (dark meat), Duck, Goose, Pheasant, Quail, Chicken (white meat), Cornish Hen, Turkey (white meat), Turkey (dark meat)

Seafood
Abalone, Anchovy, Catfish, Caviar, Clams, Crab, Crayfish, Herring, Lobster, Mackerel, Mussels, Octopus, Oysters, Perch, Pompano, Salmon, Sardines, Scallop, Shark, Shrimp, Squid, Swordfish, Trout, Tuna, Whitefish, *Bass (freshwater)*, *Bass (sea)*, *Cod*, *Grouper*, *Halibut*, *Mahi-mahi*, *Rockfish*, *Roughy*, *Snapper*

Legumes
Azuki Beans, Black Beans, Broad Beans, Butter Beans, Great Northern Beans, Green Beans, Green Peas, Kidney Beans, Lentils, Mung Beans, Navy Beans, Pink Beans, Pinto Beans, White Beans, Black-eyed Peas, Soy Beans, Tofu, Chickpeas

Beverages
Water (pure, bottled), Coffee (caffeinated), Coffee (decaf), Tea (black), Water (distilled), *Tea (green)*, *Tea (herbal)*, *Vegetable Juices*, Beer, Fruit Juices, Oat Milk, Almond Milk, Rice Milk, Soft Drinks (sodas), Soy Milk, Spirits, Water (carbonated), Water (tap), Wine (red), Wine (white)

Dairy and Eggs
Eggs, Chicken (yolks), Eggs, Duck (whole), Blue Cheese, Brie, Buttermilk, Mozzarella, Muenster, Neufchatel, Parmesan, Provolone, Colby, Cottage Cheese (low-fat), Cottage Cheese (single), Cream (single), Edam, Feta, Goat Cheese, Goat Milk, Gruyere, Ice-Cream, Milk (semi-skimmed), Milk (skimmed), Milk (whole), Monterey Jack, Ricotta, Romano, Roquefort, Sorbet, Sour-Cream, Swiss, Whey, Yogurt

Nuts and Seeds
Brazil Nuts, Filberts, Hickory Nuts, Macadamia Nuts, Peanuts, Pecans, Pumpkin Seeds, Walnuts, Almonds, Pistachios, Sesame Seeds, Cashews, Chestnuts, Pine Nuts, Poppy Seeds, Sunflower Seeds

Grains
Amaranth, Kamut, Quinoa, Spelt, Triticale, Barley, Buckwheat, Millet, Oats, Rice (basmati), Rice (brown), Rice (plain, white), Rye, Wheat, Wild Rice

Greens
Endive, Lettuce (loose-leaf), Lettuce (romaine), Lettuce (round), Radicchio, Rocket, Spinach, Spring Greens, Sprouts (alfalfa), Sprouts (bean), Turnip Greens, Watercress, Beetroot Greens, Chard, Dandelion Greens, Kale, Lettuce (iceberg), Mustard Greens

Vegetables
Artichoke, Asparagus, Avocado, Broccoli, Carrots, Cauliflower, Celery, Fennel, Garlic, Ginger Root, Jerusalem Artichoke, Leek, Mushroom (all varieties), Okra, Olive (all varieties), Onions, Radish, Shallot, Swede, Turnip, Aubergine, Bamboo Shoots, Bok Choy, Brussels Sprout, Cabbage, Courgette, Cucumber, Daikon (asian radish), Jicama, Kohlrabi, Parsnip, Pepper (bell, all colors), Pepper (hot, all colors), Pumpkin, Water Chestnuts, Beetroot, Butternut-Squash, Potato (all varieties), Squash (summer), Sweet-Potato-(yam), Sweetcorn, Tomatoes

Sea Vegetables
Agar, Dulse, Irish Moss (carrageenan), Kelp, Wakame, Laver

Fruits
Apples, Apricots, Blackberries, Blueberries, Boysenberries, Cherries, Cranberries, Elderberries, Gooseberries, Grapes, Kumquat, Loganberries, Nectarines, Papaya, Peaches, Pears, Persimmon, Plums, Raspberries, Rhubarb, Strawberries, Casaba Melon, Guava, Honeydew Melon, Kiwifruit, Mango, Pomegranate, Currants, Grapefruit, Lemons, Limes, Oranges, Prunes, Tangerines, Banana, Cantaloupe, Dates, Figs, Pineapple, Raisins, Watermelon

Oils and Fats
Borage Oil, Coconut Oil, Evening Primrose Oil, Fish Oils, Linseed Oil, Olive Oil, Palm Kernel Oil, Almond Oil, Black Currant Oil, Butter (salted), Butter (unsalted), Ghee (clarified butter), Hemp Oil, Peanut Oil, Sunflower Oil, Sesame Oil, Sunflower Oil, Wheat Germ Oil, Canola Oil, Corn Oil, Cottonseed Oil, Margarine

Herbs, Spices and Seasonings
Anise, Basil, Bay Leaf, Caraway, Cardamom, Cayenne, Chervil, Chilli Powder, Clove, Coriander, Cumin, Dill, Fennel Seed, Fenugreek, Garlic Powder, Horseradish, Mace, Marjoram, Mustard, Nutmeg, Oregano, Paprika, Peppermint, Rosemary, Saffron, Sage, Salt (sea salt, unrefined), Savory, Soy Sauce, Spearmint, Tarragon, Thyme, Turmeric, Vinegar (balsamic), Vinegar (rice), Cinnamon, Curry Powder, Ginger, Mustard Seed, Parsley, Pepper (ground black), Vanilla (extract), Carob, Mayonnaise, Molasses, Vinegar (apple cider), Wasabi, Artificial Sweeteners, Chocolate, Honey, Ketchup, Salt (iodised), Salt (low-sodium), Sugar (brown), Sugar (white), Sugar (unrefined), Vinegar (wine)

These Eating Guidelines may require modification as your health status changes. Schedule a follow-up with your practitioner.

BALANCED TYPE DIET PLAN

Eating Guidelines for Axe Adult Acne

15/04/2013

Food Colors

Green = Option #1 (eat either Option #1 or #2 at a meal, but not both)
Purple = Option #2 (eat either Option #1 or #2 at a meal, but not both)
Black = Neutral (eat freely with Option #1 or #2)
Italics = Caution (eat only rarely)
Red = Avoid (don't eat these foods)

Meats

Beef
Buffalo
Elk
Heart (beef)
Kidney (beef)
Lamb
Liver (beef)
Pork (bacon)
Rabbit
Venison
Pork (ham, chops)

Poultry

Chicken (dark meat)
Duck
Goose
Pheasant
Quail
Turkey (dark meat)
Chicken (white meat)
Cornish Hen
Turkey (white meat)

Seafood

Abalone
Anchovy
Catfish
Caviar
Clams
Crab
Crayfish
Herring
Lobster
Mackerel
Mussels
Octopus
Oysters
Perch
Pompano
Salmon
Sardines
Scallop
Shark
Shrimp
Squid
Swordfish
Trout
Tuna
Whitefish
Bass (freshwater)
Bass (sea)
Cod
Grouper
Halibut
Mahi-mahi
Rockfish
Roughy
Snapper

Legumes

Chickpeas
Navy Beans
Pink Beans
Pinto Beans
White Beans
Azuki Beans
Black Beans
Broad Beans
Butter Beans
Great Northern Beans
Green Beans
Green Peas
Kidney Beans
Lentils
Mung Beans
Black-eyed Peas
Soy Beans
Tofu

Beverages

Almond Milk
Coffee (caffeinated)
Coffee (decaf)
Oat Milk
Tea (black)
Tea (green)
Tea (herbal)
Water (distilled)
Water (pure, bottled)
Vegetable Juices
Beer
Fruit Juices
Rice Milk
Soft Drinks (colas)
Soy Milk
Spirits
Water (carbonated)
Water (tap)
Wine (red)
Wine (white)

Dairy and Eggs

Eggs, Chicken (yolks)
Eggs, Duck (whole)
Eggs, Chicken (whites)
Blue Cheese
Brie
Buttermilk
Camembert
Cheddar
Colby
Cottage Cheese
Cottage Cheese (low-fat)
Cream (single)
Cream Cheese
Edam
Feta
Goat Cheese
Goat Milk
Gouda
Gruyere
Ice Cream
Milk (semi-skimmed)
Milk (skimmed)
Milk (whole)
Monterey Jack
Mozzarella
Muenster
Neufchatel
Parmesan
Provolone
Ricotta
Romano
Roquefort
Sour Cream
Swiss
Whey
Yogurt

Nuts and Seeds

Brazil Nuts
Filberts
Hickory Nuts
Macadamia Nuts
Peanuts
Pecans
Pumpkin Seeds
Walnuts
Almonds
Cashews
Chestnuts
Pine Nuts
Pistachios
Poppy Seeds
Sesame Seeds
Sunflower Seeds

Grains

Amaranth
Kamut
Quinoa
Spelt
Triticale
Barley
Buckwheat
Millet
Oats
Rice (basmati)
Rice (brown)
Rice (plain, white)
Rye
Wheat
Wild Rice

Greens

Beetroot Greens
Chard
Coriander
Dandelion Greens
Endive
Kale
Mustard Greens
Rocket
Lettuce (iceberg)
Lettuce (loose-leaf)
Lettuce (romaine)
Lettuce (round)
Radicchio
Spinach
Spring Greens
Sprouts (alfalfa)
Sprouts (bean)
Turnip Greens
Watercress

Vegetables

Aubergine
Bamboo Shoots
Bok Choy
Broccoli
Brussels Sprout
Cabbage
Courgette
Cucumber
Daikon (asian radish)
Jicama
Kohlrabi
Parsnip
Pepper (bell, all colors)
Pepper (hot, all colors)
Pumpkin
Radish
Shallot
Winter Chestnuts
Artichoke
Asparagus
Avocado
Carrots
Cauliflower
Celery
Fennel
Garlic
Ginger Root
Jerusalem Artichoke
Leek
Mushroom (all varieties)
Okra
Olive (all varieties)
Onions
Swede
Turnip
Beetroot
Butternut Squash
Potato (white/red)
Eggplant (summer)
Sweet Potato (yam)
Sweetcorn
Tomatoes

Sea Vegetables

Dulse
Laver
Agar
Irish Moss (carrageenan)
Kelp
Wakame

Fruits

Cranberries
Elderberries
Gooseberries
Grapes
Kumquat
Loganberries
Nectarines
Peaches
Pears
Plums
Raspberries
Rhubarb
Strawberries
Currants
Grapefruit
Lemons
Limes
Oranges
Prunes
Tangerines
Banana
Cantaloupe
Dates
Figs
Pineapple
Raisins
Watermelon
Casaba Melon
Guava
Honeydew Melon
Kiwifruit
Mango
Papaya
Persimmon
Pomegranate
Apples
Apricots
Blackberries
Blueberries
Boysenberries
Cherries
Coconut

Oils and Fats

Fish Oils
Linseed Oil
Borage Oil
Coconut Oil
Evening Primrose Oil
Olive Oil
Almond Oil
Black Currant Oil
Butter (salted)
Butter (unsalted)
Ghee (clarified butter)
Hemp Oil
Peanut Oil
Safflower Oil
Sesame Oil
Sunflower Oil
Wheat Germ Oil
Canola Oil
Corn Oil
Cottonseed Oil
Margarine
Palm Kernel Oil

Herbs, Spices and Seasonings

Anise
Basil
Bay Leaf
Caraway
Cardamom
Carob
Cayenne
Chervil
Chilli Powder
Cinnamon
Cloves
Coriander
Cumin
Curry Powder
Dill
Fennel Seed
Fenugreek
Garlic Powder
Ginger
Horseradish
Mace
Marjoram
Mayonnaise
Molasses
Mustard
Mustard Seed
Nutmeg
Oregano
Paprika
Parsley
Pepper (ground black)
Peppermint
Rosemary
Saffron
Sage
Salt (sea salt, unrefined)
Savory
Soy Sauce
Spearmint
Tarragon
Thyme
Turmeric
Vanilla (extract)
Vinegar (apple cider)
Vinegar (balsamic)
Vinegar (rice)
Wasabi
Artificial Sweeteners
Chocolate
Honey
Ketchup
Salt (iodised)
Salt (low-sodium)
Sugar (brown)
Sugar (refined)
Sugar (unrefined)
Vinegar (wine)

These Eating Guidelines may require modification as your health status changes. Schedule a follow-up with your practitioner.

SLOW OXIDISER EXAMPLE DIET PLAN

Eliminate Adult Acne Four-Day Diet Plan for Slow Oxidiser – 10

	Day 1	Day 2	Day 3	Day 4
Breakfast	Soft-boiled egg(s), grapes, plum, grapefruit	Protein shake (beef collagen), coconut milk or coconut kefir, frozen blueberries, raspberries, strawberries	Poached egg, *butter*, blackberries, blueberries, strawberries, honeydew melon	Protein shake (vegetable protein), coconut milk or coconut kefir, frozen blueberries, raspberries, strawberries
Snack	Almonds & nectarine	Cashews & grapes	Pecans & strawberries	Walnuts & a plum
Lunch	Chicken soup, broccoli, cabbage, parsnip, leek, herbs	Grilled ham, *butter*, lettuce, carrot, onion, radish, red peppers, sauerkraut, olive oil & lemon juice, dried sage	Turkey soup, broccoli, cabbage, parsnip, onion, herbs	Baked wild cod, pumpkin, romaine lettuce, parsley, onion, olive oil & balsamic vinegar, steamed courgette/zucchini, dried mixed herbs
Snack				
Dinner	Grilled chicken breast, quinoa, steamed broccoli, lettuce, cucumber bell pepper, olive oil and apple cider vinegar, jerk seasoning	Pork chop, quinoa, lettuce, cucumber, celery, olive oil & apple cider vinaigrette, kimchi, fresh basil	Roasted turkey breast, lemon rub seasoning, quinoa, steamed broccoli, lettuce, spinach, cucumber, olive oil and apple cider vinegar	Wild caught Trout or Salmon, with lemon, steamed zucchini/courgette, baked pumpkin, coconut butter, lettuce, cucumber, carrot, dried oregano
Snack				

FAST OXIDISER EXAMPLE DIET PLAN

Eliminate Adult Acne Four-Day Diet Plan for Fast Oxidiser – 2O

	Day 1	Day 2	Day 3	Day 4	
Breakfast	Chicken liver pate (*butter* and 3 eggs), celery & carrot sticks	Protein shake (beef collagen), coconut water (or coconut kefir) and RO water, frozen berries, coconut oil.	Grilled bacon (nitrate-free), 3 boiled eggs, steamed asparagus, spinach.	Wild Alaskan Salmon cooked in avocado oil, poached eggs, courgette/zucchini, *mushroom*, sautéed in avocado oil, mixed herbs.	
Snack	Left over chicken pate, celery & carrot	Brazil nuts & ¼ apple	Macadamias & ¼ pear	Walnuts & blueberries	
Lunch	Roasted chicken thighs, cauliflower & carrot sauteed in *butter*, sauerkraut, jerk seasoning.	Beef stew (beef broth), artichoke & green beans sauteed in beef tallow.	Grilled pork steak, steamed carrot, spinach & kimchi, olive oil dressing, fresh oregano.	Baked wild trout, steamed broccoli & carrot, avocado oil, dried mixed herbs.	
Snack					
Dinner	Roasted chicken thighs, cauliflower & carrot sauteed in *butter*, sauerkraut, lemon chicken rub seasoning.	Beef stew (beef broth), artichoke & green beans sauteed in beef tallow.	Grilled pork steak, steamed carrot, spinach & kimchi, fresh oregano.	Baked wild trout, steamed broccoli & mushrooms, avocado oil, dried mixed herbs.	
Snack					

MIXED OXIDISER EXAMPLE DIET PLAN

Eliminate Adult Acne Four-Day Diet Plan for Mixed Oxidiser – 30

	Day 1	Day 2	Day 3	Day 4
Breakfast	Gluten-free beef burger patty, steamed kale & shallots, humous, *butter*	Freshly pressed vegetable juice (carrot, celery, turmeric), mushroom, omelette, quinoa with avocado oil	Soft boiled egg(s), nitrate-free bacon, *butter*, blueberry, raspberry, strawberry.	Protein shake (vegetable protein), coconut water and RO water, frozen blueberries, raspberries, strawberries, coconut oil.
Snack	Tahini or almond nut butter, bell peppers	½ green pear, with Brazil nuts, pecans and hazelnuts.	Boiled egg and berries (from breakfast)	½ apple, pecans, walnuts, macadamias.
Lunch	Baked wild Alaskan salmon, onion, cucumber, rocket salad, steamed zucchini/courgette, pumpkin with *ghee*, fresh oregano	*Baked cod*, steamed asparagus, cauliflower rice, sliced avocado, olive oil, lemon & herb dressing.	Chilli Con Carne, pumpkin & swede mash, rocket, cucumber, onion, bell peppers, kidney beans.	Chicken breast, artichoke, carrot, asparagus, cauliflower-rice, olive oil, jerk seasoning
Snack				
Dinner	Roast chicken thigh, onion, cucumber, rocket salad, olive oil & apple cider vinegar, parsnip with *ghee, korma masala spices*	Baked sea bass, cauliflower-rice, steamed spinach & green beans, avocado oil, basil	Roast lamb, mint, pumpkin, Steamed cabbage, *butter*, bell peppers, onion, olive oil and apple cider vinegar.	Roast chicken, quinoa, steamed asparagus & spinach, raw carrot sticks, avocado oil, garam masala spices
Snack				

SYMPATHETIC DIET PLAN

Eliminate Adult Acne Four-Day Diet Plan for Sympathetic – 1A

	Day 1	Day 2	Day 3	Day 4
Breakfast	Soft-boiled egg(s), grapefruit, apple,	Protein shake (beef collagen), coconut milk or coconut kefir and water, frozen berries	Poached egg, *butter*, blackberries, blueberries, strawberries, honeydew melon	Protein shake (vegetable protein), coconut milk and water, frozen peach & apple & mango
Snack	Almonds & apple	Cashews & grapes	Pecans & strawberries	Walnuts & a plum
Lunch	Chicken soup, broccoli, cabbage, parsnip, leek, herbs	Grilled ham, butter, lettuce, carrot, onion, radish, red peppers, sauerkraut, olive oil & lemon juice, dried sage	Turkey soup, broccoli, cabbage, parsnip, onion, herbs	Baked wild cod, pumpkin, romaine lettuce, parsley, shallot, olive oil & balsamic vinegar, steamed courgette/zucchini.
Snack				
Dinner	Grilled chicken breast, quinoa, steamed broccoli, lettuce, cucumber, bell pepper, olive oil and apple cider vinegar, jerk seasoning	Pork chop, quinoa, green leafy salad, green peppers, cucumbers, kimchi, olive oil & balsamic vinegar, dried sage	Roasted turkey breast, quinoa, steamed broccoli, lettuce, cucumber, radish, olive oil and apple cider vinegar	Wild caught Trout or Salmon, with lemon, steamed zucchini/ courgette, baked pumpkin, coconut butter, lettuce, cucumber, bell pepper, oregano
Snack				

PARASYMPATHETIC EXAMPLE DIET PLAN

Eliminate Adult Acne Four-Day Diet Plan for Parasympathetic – 2A

	Day 1	Day 2	Day 3	Day 4	
Breakfast	Chicken liver pate (*butter* and 3 eggs), celery & carrot sticks	Protein shake (beef collagen), coconut water (or coconut kefir) and RO water, frozen berries, coconut oil.	Grilled bacon (nitrate-free), 3 boiled eggs, steamed asparagus, spinach.	Wild Alaskan Salmon cooked in avocado oil, poached eggs, courgette/ zucchini, cauliflower, sautéed in avocado oil, mixed herbs.	
Snack	Left over chicken pate, celery and carrot	Brazil nuts & ¼ apple	Macadamias & ¼ pear	Walnuts & blueberries	
Lunch	Roasted chicken thighs, cauliflower & carrot sauteed in *butter*, sauerkraut, jerk seasoning.	Beef stew (beef broth), leek & green beans sauteed in beef tallow.	Grilled pork steak, steamed asparagus, spinach & sauerkraut, fresh oregano.	Baked wild trout, steamed broccoli & *mushrooms*, avocado oil, dried mixed herbs.	
Snack					
Dinner	Roasted chicken thighs, cauliflower & carrot sauteed in *butter*, sauerkraut, lemon rub seasoning.	Beef stew (beef broth), leek & green beans sauteed in beef tallow.	Grilled pork steak, steamed asparagus, spinach & kimchi, fresh oregano.	Baked wild trout, steamed broccoli & *mushrooms*, avocado oil, dried mixed herbs.	
Snack					

BALANCED TYPE EXAMPLE DIET PLAN

Eliminate Adult Acne Four-Day Diet Plan for Balanced – 3A

	Day 1	Day 2	Day 3	Day 4
Breakfast	Gluten-free beef burger patty, steamed kale & shallots, humous, *butter*	Freshly pressed vegetable juice (carrot, celery, ginger), mushroom-omelette, quinoa with avocado oil	Soft boiled egg(s), bacon, *butter*, Kiwifruit, mango, papaya.	Protein shake (vegetable protein), coconut water or coconut kefir, frozen blueberries, raspberries, strawberries, coconut oil.
Snack	Tahini or almond nut butter, cucumber sticks	½ green pear, almonds, cashews & pistachios.	Boiled egg and fruit (from breakfast)	½ apple, almonds, cashews and pine nuts.
Lunch	Baked wild Alaskan salmon, pumpkin with *ghee*, cucumber, rocket & shallot salad, steamed zucchini/courgette, dried oregano	*Baked sea bass*, quinoa, steamed asparagus, sliced avocado, olive oil, lemon & herb dressing.	Chilli Con Carne, parsnip and pumpkin mash with *ghee*, rocket, cucumber, bell peppers, shallot, kidney beans.	Chicken breast, artichoke, carrot, asparagus, cauliflower-rice, sauerkraut, olive oil, Italian seasoning
Snack				
Dinner	Roast lamb, mint, parsnip with *ghee*, cucumber, rocket & shallot salad, olive oil & apple cider vinegar	Baked cod, avocado, cauliflower-rice, steamed spinach & green beans with avocado oil, fresh parsley	Beef liver, pumpkin, Steamed cabbage, *butter*, bell peppers, shallot, olive oil and apple cider vinegar.	Roast chicken, quinoa, steamed asparagus & spinach, raw carrot sticks, kimchi, avocado oil, garam masala spice mix
Snack				

4-DAY DIET PLAN TEMPLATE

Day 1	Day 2	Day 3	Day 4
Breakfast:	Breakfast:	Breakfast:	Breakfast:
Snack:	Snack:	Snack:	Snack:
Lunch:	Lunch:	Lunch:	Lunch:
Snack:	Snack:	Snack:	Snack:
Dinner:	Dinner:	Dinner:	Dinner:

PULSE TESTING SHEET

Food Item or Supplement	Pre-test Pulse Rate	Post-test Pulse Rate	Difference in Beats Per Minute (= or > +/- 4)

GENERIC ACNE DIET PLAN

8/3/2011

Eating Guidelines for Ann Example

Food Colors

Green = Ideal (eat ideal foods at every meal)
Black = Neutral (ok, but emphasize "Ideal" foods)
Italics = Caution (eat rarely or only for variety)
Red = Avoid (don't eat these foods)

Meats
Beef, Buffalo, Elk, Heart (beef), Kidney (beef), Lamb, Liver (beef), Pork (ham, chops), Rabbit, Venison, Pork (bacon)

Poultry
Chicken (dark meat), Duck, Goose, Quail, Turkey (dark meat), Chicken (white meat), Cornish Hen, Pheasant, Turkey (white meat)

Seafood
Anchovy, Bass (freshwater), Bass (sea), Catfish, Caviar, Clams, Crab, Halibut, Herring, Lobster, Mackerel, Mussels, Octopus, Oysters, Perch, Pompano, Rockfish, Salmon, Sardines, Scallop, Shark, Shrimp, Snapper, Squid, Swordfish, Trout, Tuna, Whitefish, Abalone, Cod, Crayfish, Grouper, Mahi-mahi, Roughy

Legumes
Soy Beans, Tofu, Azuki Beans, Black Beans, Fava Beans, Garbanzo Beans, Great Northern Beans, Green Beans, Green Peas, Lentils, Lima Beans, Mung Beans, Navy Beans, Pink Beans, Pinto Beans, Red Beans, White Beans, Black-eyed Peas

Beverages
Water (tap), Beer, Fruit Juices, Liquor, Rice Milk, Soft Drinks (colas), Wine (red), Wine (white), Almond Milk, Coffee (caffeinated), Coffee (decaf), Oat Milk, Soy Milk, Tea (black), Tea (green), Tea (herbal), Vegetable Juices, Water (carbonated), Water (distilled), Water (pure, bottled)

Dairy and Eggs
Eggs, Chicken (yolks), Eggs, Duck (whole), Eggs, Chicken (whites), Blue-Cheese, Brie, Buttermilk, Camembert, Cheddar, Colby, Cottage-Cheese (late), Cottage-Cheese (skim), Cream-Cheese (half-and-half), Cream-Cheese, Edam, Feta, Goat-Cheese, Goat-Milk, Gouda, Gruyere, Ice-Cream, Milk (2%), Milk (skim), Milk (whole), Monterrey-Jack, Muenster, Neufchatel, Provolone, Ricotta, Romano, Roquefort, Sorbet, Sour-Cream, Swiss, Whey, Yogurt

Nuts and Seeds
Hickory Nuts, Pecans, Pine Nuts, Pumpkin Seeds, Walnuts, Almonds, Brazil Nuts, Cashews, Chestnuts, Filberts, Macadamia Nuts, Peanuts, Pistachios, Poppy Seeds, Sesame Seeds, Sunflower Seeds

Grains
Amaranth, Kamut, Quinoa, Spelt, Triticale, Barley, Buckwheat, Millet, Oats, Rice (basmati), Rice (brown), Rice (plain, white), Rye, Wheat, Wild-Rice

Greens
Arugula, Endive, Watercress, Beet Greens, Cilantro, Collard Greens, Dandelion Greens, Kale, Lettuce (bibb), Lettuce (iceberg), Lettuce (loose-leaf), Lettuce (romaine), Mustard Greens, Radicchio, Spinach, Sprouts (alfalfa), Sprouts (bean), Swiss Chard, Turnip Greens

Vegetables
Asparagus, Broccoli, Carrots, Shallot, Artichoke, Avocado, Bamboo Shoots, Bok Choy, Brussels Sprout, Cabbage, Cauliflower, Celery, Cucumber, Daikon, Eggplant, Fennel, Garlic, Ginger Root, Jerusalem Artichoke, Jicama, Kohlrabi, Mushroom (all varieties), Okra, Olive (all varieties), Onions, Parsnip, Pepper (bell, all colors), Pepper (hot, all colors), Pumpkin, Radish, Rutabaga, Turnip, Water Chestnuts, Zucchini, Beets, Gem, Potato (all varieties), Squash (summer), Squash (winter), Sweet-Potato (yam), Tomatoes

Sea Vegetables
Dulse, Agar, Irish Moss (carrageenan), Kelp, Laver, Wakame

Fruits
Apricots, Cherries, Grapefruit, Papaya, Persimmon, Apples, Blackberries, Blueberries, Boysenberries, Casaba Melon, Coconut, Cranberries, Currants, Elderberries, Gooseberries, Grapes, Guava, Honeydew Melon, Kiwifruit, Kumquat, Lemons, Limes, Loganberries, Mango, Nectarines, Oranges, Peaches, Pears, Plums, Pomegranate, Prunes, Raspberries, Rhubarb, Strawberries, Tangerines, Banana, Cantaloupe, Dates, Figs, Pineapple, Raisins, Watermelon

Oils and Fats
Black Currant Oil, Canola Oil, Fish Oils, Flaxseed Oil, Hemp Oil, Wheat Germ Oil, Almond Oil, Borage Oil, Coconut Oil, Corn Oil, Cottonseed Oil, Evening Primrose Oil, Olive Oil, Palm Kernel Oil, Peanut Oil, Safflower Oil, Sesame Oil, Sunflower Oil, Butter (salted), Butter (unsalted), Ghee (clarified butter), Margarine

Herbs, Spices and Seasonings
Anise, Artificial Sweeteners, Basil, Bay Leaf, Caraway, Cardamom, Carob, Cayenne, Chervil, Chili Powder, Chive, Cinnamon, Cloves, Coriander, Cumin, Curry Powder, Dill Weed, Fennel Seed, Fenugreek, Garlic Powder, Ginger, Horseradish, Mace, Marjoram, Mayonnaise, Molasses, Mustard, Mustard Seed, Nutmeg, Oregano, Paprika, Parsley, Pepper (ground black), Peppermint, Rosemary, Saffron, Sage, Salt (iodized), Salt (low sodium), Salt (sea salt, unrefined), Savory, Soy Sauce, Spearmint, Tarragon, Thyme, Turmeric, Vanilla (extract), Vinegar (apple cider), Vinegar (balsamic), Vinegar (rice), Vinegar (wine), Wasabi, Chocolate, Honey, Ketchup, Sugar (brown), Sugar (white), Sugar (brown, unrefined)

These Eating Guidelines may require modification as your health status changes. Schedule a follow-up with your practitioner.

RESOURCES

1. For most of the resources required when following this programme, please go to https://eliminateadultacne.com/resources.

2. If you require professional help when implementing this programme, I do have a coaching programme called Eliminate Adult Acne, the details of which can be found at https://skinwebinar.com.

3. Instructions for the online Metabolic Typing® Test are available at https://eliminateadultacne.com/resources.

4. *The Metabolic Typing Diet*, by William Wolcott and Trish Fahey (2002).

5. You can check the safety/toxicity levels of your personal care products at https://www.ewg.org/skindeep/.

6. My podcast, *The Radical Health Rebel,* where I discuss a number of health subjects every week, including acne, can be found at http://radicalhealthrebel.com and all major podcast platforms.

7. Good quality dietary supplement sites:
   a. https://synergisticseurope.com (Use Code LB753) (UK/EU)
   b. https://www.ultralifeinc.com (USA)
   c. https://invivohealthcare.com/products/supplements/ (UK/EU)
   d. https://bit.ly/WelldiumAcne (EU)
   e. https://bit.ly/KiScienceProducts (UK)
   f. https://planetpaleo.co - 10% Discount Code 'LEIGH67640' (UK)
   g. https://bioptimizers.uk/radicalrebel

REFERENCES

Acromegaly. (n.d.). Merriam-Webster Dictionary. https://www.merriam-webster.com/dictionary/acromegaly

Akaza, N., Akamatsu, H., Numata, S., Yamada, S., Yagami, A., Nakata, S. and Matsunaga, K. (2016). Microorganisms inhabiting follicular contents of facial acne are not only Propionibacterium but also Malassezia spp. *J Dermatol*, 43, 906-911.

Akaza, N., Akamatsu, H., Takeoka, S., Sasaki, Y., Mizutani, H., Nakata, S. and Matsunaga, K. (2012). *Malassezia* globosa tends to grow actively in summer conditions more than other cutaneous *Malassezia* species. *J Dermatol*, 39, 613-616.

Ali, S.M. & Yosipovitch, G. (2013). Skin pH: From Basic SciencE to Basic Skin Care. *Acta Dermato-Venereologica*, 93(3), 261-267. https://doi.org/10.2340/00015555-1531

Anoxic. (n.d.). Merriam-Webster Dictionary. https://www.merriam-webster.com/dictionary/anoxic

Asha, M.K., Debraj, D., Dethe, S., Bhaskar, A., Muruganantham, N. and Deepak, M. (2017, May 4). Effect of Flavonoid-Rich Extract of Glycyrrhiza glabra on Gut-Friendly Microorganisms, Commercial Probiotic Preparations, and Digestive Enzymes. *J Diet Suppl,* 14(3), 323-333. DOI: 10.1080/19390211.2016.1223257.

Basmatker, G., Jains, N. and Daud, F. (2011) Aloe vera: a valuable multifunctional cosmetic ingredient. *International Journal of Medicinal and Aromatic Plants*, 1, 338-341./

Bhat. Y.J., Latief, I. and Hassan, I. (2017, May-June). Update on etiopathogenesis and treatment of Acne. *Indian J Dermatol Venereol Leprol*, 83(3), 298-306. DOI: 10.4103/0378-6323.199581.

Biomatrix Quick Reference Chart. (2000). BioHealth Diagnostics, Inc. http://biodia.com/biomatrix/biomatrix.htm

Blaak, J., Dähnhardt, D., Dähnhardt-Pfeiffer, S., Bielfeldt, S., Wilhelm, K.P., Wohlfart, R. and Staib, P. (2017). A plant oil-containing pH 4 emulsion improves epidermal barrier structure and enhances ceramide levels in aged skin. *Int J Cosmet Sci*, 39, 284-291. https://doi.org/10.1111/ics.12374

Borgia, F., Cannavò, S., Guarneri, F., Cannavò, SP., Vaccaro, M., and Guarneri, B. (2004). Correlation between endocrinological parameters and acne severity in adult women. *Acta Derm Venereol*, 84(3), 201-24. DOI: 10.1080/00015550410023248

Bouwstra, J.A., Ponec, M. (2006, December). The skin barrier in healthy and diseased state. *Biochim Biophys Acta*, 1758(12), 2080-2095. DOI: 10.1016/j.bbamem.2006.06.021

Bowe, W.P. and Logan, A.C. (2011, January 31). Acne vulgaris, probiotics and the gut-brain-skin axis - back to the future? *Gut Pathog*, 3(1), 1. DOI: 10.1186/1757-4749-3-1.

Brackett, C. and Waldron, J.T. (Directors). (2014, September 14). *Sweet Misery: A Poisoned World* [Film]. Video Service Corp.

Bures, J., Cyrany, J., Kohoutova, D., Förstl, M., Rejchrt, S., Kvetina, J., Vorisek, V. and Kopacova, M. (2010, June 28). Small intestinal bacterial overgrowth syndrome. *World J Gastroenterol*, 16(24), 2978-2990. DOI: 10.3748/wjg.v16.i24.2978.

Byrd, A., Belkaid, Y. and Segre, J. (2018). The human skin microbiome. *Nat Rev Microbiol*, 16, 143-155. https://doi.org/10.1038/nrmicro.2017.157

Çerman, A.A., Aktaş, E., Altunay, İ.K., Arıcı, J.E., Tulunay, A. and Ozturk, F.Y. (2016, July). Dietary glycemic factors, insulin resistance, and adiponectin levels in acne vulgaris. *J Am Acad Dermatol*, 75(1), 155-162. DOI: 10.1016/j.jaad.2016.02.1220.

Chek, P. (2004, February 7). *How To Eat, Move And Be Healthy*. Carlsbad: CHEK Institute.

Chen, K., Xie, K., Liu, Z., Nakasone, Y., Sakao, K., Hossain, A. and Hou, D.X. (2019, May 29). Preventive Effects and Mechanisms of Garlic on Dyslipidemia and Gut Microbiome Dysbiosis. *Nutrients*, 11(6), 1225. doi: 10.3390/nu11061225.

Chen, Q., Chen, O., Martins, I.M., Hou, H., Zhao, X., Blumberg, J.B. and Li, B. (2017, March 22). Collagen peptides ameliorate intestinal epithelial barrier dysfunction in immunostimulatory Caco-2 cell monolayers via enhancing tight junctions. *Food Funct*, 8(3), 1144-1151. DOI: 10.1039/c6fo01347c.

Combined Pill: Your Contraceptive Guide. (2020, July 1). NHS. https://www.nhs.uk/conditions/contraception/combined-contraceptive-pill

Commensal. (n.d.). Merriam-Webster Dictionary. https://www.merriam-webster.com/dictionary/commensal

Cordain, L., Lindeberg, S., Hurtado, M., Hill, K., Eaton, S.B., and Brand-Miller, J. (2002, December). Acne vulgaris: a disease of Western civilization. *Arch Dermatol*, 138(12), 1584-1590. DOI: 10.1001/archderm.138.12.1584.

Costinescu, S. (2009, September 2). *Pharmafia's Top 10 Biggest Healthcare Fraud Fines in US History*. Silview. https://silview.media/2021/07/22/pharmafias-top-10-biggest-healthcare-fraud-fines/

Cordain, L., Eades, M.R., and Eades, M.D. (2003, September). Hyperinsulinemic diseases of civilization: more than just Syndrome X. *Comp Biochem Physiol A Mol Integr Physiol*, 136(1), 95-112. DOI: 10.1016/s1095-6433(03)00011-4

Cytosol. (n.d.). Merriam-Webster Dictionary. https://www.merriam-webster.com/dictionary/cytosol

Danby, F.W. (2013, July). Turning acne on/off via mTORC1. *Exp Dermatol*, 22(7), 505-506. DOI: 10.1111/exd.12180.

Danby, F.W. (2010, November-December). Nutrition and acne. *Clin Dermatol*, 28(6), 598-604. DOI: 10.1016/j.clindermatol.2010.03.017

Darley, C.R., Moore, J.W., Besser, G.M., Munro, D.D., Edwards, C.R., Rees, L.H. and Kirby, J.D. (1984, January). Androgen status in women with late onset or persistent acne vulgaris. *Clin Exp Dermatol*, 9(1), 28-35. DOI: 10.1111/j.1365-2230.1984.tb00751.x.

Demasi, M. (2022, June 29). From FDHA to MHRA: are drug regulators for hire? *BMJ*, 377. DOI: https://doi.org/10.1136/bmj.o1538

Deutsch, R. and Rivera R. (2002, July 23). *Your Hidden Food Allergies Are Making You Fat, Revised: How to Lose Weight and Gain Years of Vitality*. Roseville: Prima.

Dgotto. (2006, November 15). *mTor exists in at least two distinct protein complexes* [Image]. mTOR: growth regulator involved in disease. Slideshare. https://image.slidesharecdn.com/mtor-growth-regulator-involved-in-disease-14262/95/mtor-growth-regulator-involved-in-disease-7728.jpg?cb=1163582983

Doctors turning to antibiotic alternatives to treat acne. (2019, April 24). Science Daily. https://www.sciencedaily.com/releases/2019/04/190424125214.htm

Electrical Sensitivity—What's It All About? (2014, July 8). The Healthy House. https://healthy-house.co.uk/allergy-blog/electrical-sensitivity-whats-it-all-about/

Enzyme. (2001, September 29). Wikipedia. https://en.wikipedia.org/wiki/Enzyme

Eo, J., Seo, Y.K., Baek, J.H., Choi, A.R., Shin, M.K. and Koh, J.S. (2016). Facial skin physiology recovery kinetics during 180 min postwashing with a cleanser. *Skin Res Technol*, 22: 148-151. https://doi.org/10.1111/srt.12241

Epithelium. (n.d.). Merriam-Webster Dictionary. https://www.merriam-webster.com/dictionary/epithelium

Essential Oils Desk Reference. (2000, January 1). Draper: Essential Science Publishing.

Find Drugs & Conditions. (n.d.). Drugs.com. https://www.drugs.com/

Finlay, B. and Finlay, J. (2019). *The Whole-Body Microbiome.* New York: The Experiment Publishing.

Frasca, G., Cardile, V., Puglia, C., Bonina, C. and Bonina, F. (2012, May 8). Gelatin tannate reduces the proinflammatory effects of lipopolysaccharide in human intestinal epithelial cells. *Clin Exp Gastroenterol*, 5, 61-67. DOI: 10.2147/CEG.S28792.

Grice, E.A. and Segre, J.A. (2011, April). The skin microbiome. *Nat Rev Microbiol*, 9(4), 244-53. DOI: 10.1038/nrmicro2537.

Gorbach, S.L. (1993). Perturbation of intestinal microflora. *Vet Hum Toxicol*, 35 Suppl 1, 15-23. PMID: 7901933

Gorbach, S.L., Barza, M., Giuliano, M. and Jacobus, N.V. (1988). Colonization resistance of the human intestinal microflora: Testing the hypothesis in normal volunteers. *Eur. J. Clin. Microbiol. Infect. Dis.*, 7, 98–102. https://doi.org/10.1007/BF01962192

Goulden, V., McGeown, C.H. and Cunliffe, W.J. (1999, August). The familial risk of adult acne: a comparison between first-degree relatives of affected and unaffected individuals. *Br J Dermatol*, 141(2), 297-300. DOI: 10.1046/j.1365-2133.1999.02979.x.

Greenberg, J. (2021, June 16). *Naturopathic and Integrative Dermatology Series: The mTOR Pathway and Acne: Linking Nutrition to Biochemistry*. Learnskin. https://www.learnskin.com/courses/naturopathy/the-mtor-pathway-and-acne-linking-nutrition-to-biochemistry

Hawrelak, J. & Myers, S. (2004). The causes of intestinal dysbiosis: A review. *Alternative medicine review: a journal of clinical therapeutic*, 9, 180-197.

Hu, G., Wei, Y.P. and Feng, J. (2010). Malassezia infection: is there any chance or necessity in refractory acne? *Chin Med J (Engl)*, 123, 628-632.

Huang, J.Y., Sweeney, E.G., Guillemin, K. and Amieva, M.R. (2017, January 19). Multiple Acid Sensors Control Helicobacter pylori Colonization of the Stomach. *PLoS Pathog*, 13(1), e1006118. DOI: 10.1371/journal.ppat.1006118.

Immune System. (2001, September 4) Wikipedia. https://en.wikipedia.org/wiki/Immune_system

Isotretinoin capsules (Roaccutane). (2022, February 28). NHS. https://www.nhs.uk/medicines/isotretinoin-capsules/

Jang, H., Matsuda, A., Jung, K., Karasawa, K., Matsuda, K., Oida, K., Ishizaka, S., Ahn, G., Amagai, Y., Moon, C., Kim, S., Arkwright, P.D., Takamori, K., Matsuda, H. and Tanaka, A. (2016, January). Skin pH Is Skin pH Is the Master Switch of Kallikrein 5-Mediated Skin Barrier Destruction in a Murine Atopic Dermatitis Model. *Journal of Investigative Dermatology*, 136(1), 127-135. https://doi.org/10.1038/JID.2015.363SDFSDF

Ju, Q., Tao, T., Hu, T., Karadağ, A.S., Al-Khuzaei, S. and Chen, W. (2017, March-April). Sex hormones and acne. *Clin Dermatol*, 35(2), 130-137. DOI: 10.1016/j.clindermatol.2016.10.004.

Jung, J.Y., Yoon, M.Y., Min, S.U., Hong, J.S., Choi, Y.S., and Suh, D.H. (2010, November-December). The influence of dietary patterns on acne vulgaris in Koreans. *Eur J Dermatol*, 20(6), 768-772. DOI: 10.1684/ejd.2010.1053

Kakiyama, G., Pandak, W.M., Gillevet, P.M., Hylemon, P.B., Heuman, D.M., Daita, K., Takei, H., Muto, A., Nittono, H., Ridlon, J.M., White, M.B., Noble, N.A., Monteith, P., Fuchs, M., Thacker, L.R., Sikaroodi, M. and Bajaj, J.S. (2013, May). Modulation of the fecal bile acid profile by gut microbiota in cirrhosis. *J Hepatol*, 58(5), 949-955. DOI: 10.1016/j.jhep.2013.01.003.

Katsuta, Y., Iida, T., Inomata, S. and Denda M. (2005). Unsaturated fatty acids induce calcium influx into keratinocytes and cause abnormal differentiation of epidermis. *J Invest Dermatol*, 124, 1008-1013.

Kennedy, R.F. Jr. (2021, November 16). *The Real Anthony Fauci: Bill Gates, Big Pharma, and the Global War on Democracy and Public Health*. New York: Skyhorse Publishing.

Keratin. (n.d.). Merriam-Webster Dictionary. https://www.merriam-webster.com/dictionary/keratin

Keratinocyte. (n.d.) Merriam-Webster Dictionary. https://www.merriam-webster.com/dictionary/keratinocyte

Kesavan, S., Walters, C.E., Holland, K.T. and Ingham. E. (1998). The effects of Malassezia on pro-inflammatory cytokine production by human peripheral blood mononuclear cells in vitro. *Med Mycol*, 36, 97-106.

Khan, H. and Thomas, P. (2010, April 17). *Drug Giant AstraZeneca to Pay $520 Million to Settle Fraud Case Government says pharmaceutical firm illegally marketed schizophrenia drug*. ABC News. https://abcnews.go.com/Politics/Health/astrazeneca-pay-520-million-illegally-marketing-seroquel-schizophrenia/story?id=10488647

Miller, C.S. and Ashford, N.A. (1990). *Chemical Exposures: Low Levels and High Stakes*, K.H. Kilburn (Ed.). New York: Van Nostrand Reinhold,

Kim, E., Kim, S., Nam, G.W., Lee, H., Moon, S. and Chang, I. (2009), The alkaline pH-adapted skin barrier is disrupted severely by SLS-induced irritation. *International Journal of Cosmetic Science*, 31: 263-269. https://doi.org/10.1111/j.1468-2494.2009.00491.x

Kim, K.P., Jeon, S., Kim, M.J. and Cho, Y. (2018b, October). Borage oil restores acidic skin pH by up-regulating the activity or expression of filaggrin and enzymes involved in epidermal lactate, free fatty acid, and acidic free amino acid metabolism in essential fatty acid-deficient Guinea pigs. *Nutr Res*, 58, 26-35. DOI: 10.1016/j.nutres.2018.06.003.

Kim, K., Jeon, S., Kim, M., Cho, Y. (2018). Borage oil restores acidic skin pH by up-regulating the activity or expression of filaggrin and enzymes involved in epidermal lactate, free fatty acid, and acidic free amino acid metabolism in essential fatty acid-deficient Guinea pigs. *Nutrition Research*, 58, 2018, 26-35. https://doi.org/10.1016/j.nutres.2018.06.003

Kingston, K. (2023, January 15). *The hidden risks of electric blankets.* Karen Kingston's Blog. https://www.karenkingston.com/blog/electric-blankets/

Klinghardt, D. (2020, July). Klinghardt Institute Summer School.

Kober, M.M. and Bowe, W.P. (2015, April 6). The effect of probiotics on immune regulation, acne, and photoaging. *Int J Womens Dermatol,* 1(2), 85-89. doi: 10.1016/j.ijwd.2015.02.001.

Korting, H.C., Kerscher, M., Schäfer-Korting, M. and Berchtenbreiter, U. (1993). Influence of topical erythromycin preparations for acne vulgaris on skin surface pH. *Clin Investig* 71, 644-648. https://doi.org/10.1007/BF00184493

Laplante, M. and Sabatini, D.M. (2009, October 15). mTOR signaling at a glance. *J Cell Sci,* 122(Pt 20), 3589-3594. DOI: 10.1242/jcs.051011.

Larch Arabinogalactan—Uses, Side Effects, and More. (n.d.). Web MD. https://www.webmd.com/vitamins/ai/ingredientmono-974/larch-arabinogalactan

Leading Lobbying industries in the United States in 2022, by total lobbying spending(in million U.S. dollars). (2023). Statista. https://www.statista.com/statistics/257364/top-lobbying-industries-in-the-us/

Lee, Y.B., Byun, E.J. and Kim, H.S. (2019, July 7). Potential Role of the Microbiome in Acne: A Comprehensive Review. *J Clin Med*, 8(7), 987. DOI: 10.3390/jcm8070987.

Leo, M.S. and Sivamani, R.K. (2014, December). Phytochemical modulation of the Akt/mTOR pathway and its potential use in cutaneous disease. *Arch Dermatol Res*, 306(10). 861-871. DOI: 10.1007/s00403-014-1480-8.

Li. T. and Wang G. (2014, October 20). Computer-aided targeting of the PI3K/Akt/mTOR pathway: toxicity reduction and therapeutic opportunities. *Int J Mol Sci*, 15(10), 18856-18891. DOI: 10.3390/ijms151018856.

Lipophilic. (n.d.). Merriam-Webster Dictionary. https://www.merriam-webster.com/dictionary/lipophilic

Lizasa, H., Ishihara, S., Richardo, T., Kanehiro, Y. and Yoshiyama, H. (2015, October 28). Dysbiotic infection in the stomach. *World J Gastroenterol*, 21(40), 11450-11457. DOI: 10.3748/wjg.v21.i40.11450.

Luebberding, S., Krueger, N. and Kerscher, M. (2013). Skin physiology in men and women: *in vivo*evaluation of 300 people including TEWL, SC hydration, sebum content and skin surface pH. *Int J Cosmet Sci*, 35: 477-483. https://doi.org/10.1111/ics.12068

Mani, V., Hollis, J.H. and Gabler, N.K. (2013, January 10). Dietary oil composition differentially modulates intestinal endotoxin transport and postprandial endotoxemia. *Nutr Metab (Lond)*, 10(1), 6. DOI: 10.1186/1743-7075-10-6.

Marchetti, F., Capizzi, R. and Tulli, A. (1987, September 15). Efficacia dei regolatori della flora batterica intestinale nella terapia dell'acne volgare [Efficacy of regulators of the intestinal bacterial flora in the therapy of acne vulgaris]. *Clin Ter*, 122(5), 339-343. PMID: 2972450.

Melnik, B.C. (2018, January-February). Acne vulgaris: The metabolic syndrome of the pilosebaceous follicle. *Clin Dermatol*, 36(1), 29-40. DOI: 10.1016/j.clindermatol.2017.09.006.

Melnik, B.C. (2017, March). The TRAIL to acne pathogenesis: let's focus on death pathways. *Exp Dermatol*, 26(3), 270-272. DOI: 10.1111/exd.13169.

Melnik, B.C. and Schmitz, G. (2013, July). Are therapeutic effects of antiacne agents mediated by activation of FoxO1 and inhibition of mTORC1? *Exp Dermatol*, 22(7), 502-504. DOI: 10.1111/exd.12172.

Melnik, B.C. and Zouboulis, C.C. (2013, May). Potential role of FoxO1 and mTORC1 in the pathogenesis of Western diet-induced acne. *Exp Dermatol*, 22(5), 311-315. DOI: 10.1111/exd.12142.

Melnik, B.C. (2012, May). Diet in acne: further evidence for the role of nutrient signalling in acne pathogenesis. *Acta Derm Venereol*, 92(3), 228-231. DOI: 10.2340/00015555-1358.

Melnik, B.C. (2011). Evidence for acne-promoting effects of milk and other insulinotropic dairy products. *Nestle Nutr Workshop Ser Pediatr Program*, 67, 131-145. DOI: 10.1159/000325580

Menon, D., Salloum, D., Bernfeld, E., Gorodetsky, E., Akselrod. A., Frias, M.A., Sudderth. J., Chen. P.H., DeBerardinis, R. and Foster, D.A. (2017, April 14). Lipid sensing by mTOR complexes via de novo synthesis of phosphatidic acid. *J Biol Chem*, 292(15), 6303-6311. DOI: 10.1074/jbc.M1

Michielan, A. and D'Incà, R. (2015). Intestinal Permeability in Inflammatory Bowel Disease: Pathogenesis, Clinical Evaluation, and Therapy of Leaky Gut. *Mediators Inflamm.* DOIL 10.1155/2015/628157.

Microbiota. (n.d.). Merriam-Webster Dictionary. https://www.merriam-webster.com/dictionary/microbiota

Monfrecola, G., Lembo, S., Caiazzo, G., De Vita, V., Di Caprio, R., Balato, A. and Fabbrocini, G. (2016), Mechanistic target of rapamycin (mTOR) expression is increased in acne patients' skin. *Exp Dermatol*, 25, 153-155. https://doi.org/10.1111/exd.12885

Mucin. (2004, December 1). Wikipedia. https://en.wikipedia.org/wiki/Mucin

Mudgil. D., Barak, S., Patel, A. and Shah, N. (2018, June). Partially hydrolyzed guar gum as a potential prebiotic source. *Int J Biol Macromol*, 112, 207-210. doi: 10.1016/j.ijbiomac.2018.01.164.

Numata, S., Akamatsu, H., Akaza, N., Yagami, A., Nakata, S. and Matsunaga, K. (2014). Analysis of facial skin-resident microbiota in Japanese acne patients. *Dermatology,* 228, 86-92.

O'Neill, C.A., Monteleone, G., McLaughlin, J.T. and Paus, R. (2016, November). The gut-skin axis in health and disease: A paradigm with therapeutic implications. *Bioessays*, 38(11), 1167-1176. DOI: 10.1002/bies.201600008

Osmosis Beauty. (2020, January 30). *Osmosis Beauty- Understanding The Relationship: Dairy and Acne* [Video]. YouTube. https://www.youtube.com/watch?v=Yqd5EixfV54

Overview: Acne. (2017, September 21). NHS. https://www.nhs.uk/conditions/acne/

Pathogen. (n.d.). Merriam-Webster Dictionary. https://www.merriam-webster.com/dictionary/pathogen

Pert, C. (1999, February 17). *Molecules of Emotion: The Science Behind Mind-Body Medicine.* New York: Scribner.

Pfizer to pay record $2.3 billion penalty. (2009, September 2). NBC News. https://www.nbcnews.com/id/wbna32657347

pH. (2001, October 31). Wikipedia. https://en.wikipedia.org/wiki/PH

Phosphorylate. (n.d.). Merriam-Webster dictionary. https://www.merriam-webster.com/dictionary/phosphorylate

Pochi, P.E. (1982, August). Acne: endocrinologic aspects. *Cutis*, 30(2), 212-214, 216-217, 219 passim. PMID: 6215213

Polychlorinated biphenyl. (n.d.). Merrian-Webster Dictionary. https://www.merriam-webster.com/dictionary/polychlorinated%20biphenyl

Prakash, C., Bhargava, P., Tiwari, S., Majumdar, B. and Bhargava, R.K. (2017, July). Skin Surface pH in Acne Vulgaris: Insights from an Observational Study and Review of the Literature. *J Clin Aesthet Dermatol*, 10(7), 33-39. PMID: 29104722; PMCID: PMC5605222.

Proksch, E. (2018). pH in nature, humans and skin. *J Dermatol*, 45, 1044-1052. https://doi.org/10.1111/1346-8138.14489

Pugh, J.N., Sage, S., Hutson, M., Doran, D.A., Fleming, S.C., Highton, J., Morton, J.P. and Close, G.L. (2017, December). Glutamine supplementation reduces markers of intestinal permeability during running in the heat in a dose-dependent manner. *Eur J Appl Physiol*, 117(12), 2569-2577. DOI: 10.1007/s00421-017-3744-4.

Rivera, R. & Deutsch, R. (1998, August 31). *Your Hidden Food Allergies Are Making You Fat: The ALCAT Test Weight Loss Breakthrough.* Toronto: Prima.

Rusu, E., Enache, G., Cursaru, R., Alexescu, A., Radu, R., Onila, O., Cavallioti, T., Rusu, F., Posea, M., Jinga, M. and Radulian, G. (2019,

August). Prebiotics and probiotics in atopic dermatitis. *Exp Ther Med*, 18(2), 926-931. doi: 10.3892/etm.2019.7678.

Salem, I., Ramser, A., Isham, N., Ghannoum, M.A. (2018, July 10). The Gut Microbiome as a Major Regulator of the Gut-Skin Axis. *Front Microbiol*, 9, 1459. DOI: 10.3389/fmicb.2018.01459. PMID: 30042740

Sansone, G. and Reisner, R.M. (1971, May). Differential rates of conversion of testosterone to dihydrotestosterone in acne and in normal human skin—a possible pathogenic factor in acne. *J Invest Dermatol*, 56(5), 366-372. DOI: 10.1111/1523-1747.ep12261252.

Scourboutakos, M.J., Franco-Arellano, B., Murphy, S.A., Norsen, S., Comelli, E.M. and L'Abbé, M.R. (2017, April 18). Mismatch between Probiotic Benefits in Trials versus Food Products. *Nutrients*. doi: 10.3390/nu9040400.

Sebum. (n.d.). Merrium-Webster Dictionary. https://www.merriam-webster.com/dictionary/sebum

Segre, J.A. (2006, May). Epidermal barrier formation and recovery in skin disorders. *J Clin Invest*, 116(5), 1150-1158. DOI: 10.1172/JCI28521.

Shen, L., Liu, L. and Ji, H.F. (2017, August 9). Regulative effects of curcumin spice administration on gut microbiota and its pharmacological implications. *Food Nutr Res*, 61(1), e1361780. DOI: 10.1080/16546628.2017.1361780.

Side effects of spironolactone—Brand name: Aldactone. (2022, July 8). NHS. https://www.nhs.uk/medicines/spironolactone/side-effects-of-spironolactone/

Slayden, S.M., Moran, C., Sams, W.M. Jr., Boots, L.R., and Aziz, R. (2001, May). Hyperandrogenemia in patients presenting with acne. *Fertil Steril*, 75(5), 1-701. DOI: 10.1016/s0015-0282(01)01701-0

Sloan, T.J., Jalanka, J., Major, G.A.D., Krishnasamy, S., Pritchard, S., Abdelrazig, S., Korpela, K., Singh, G., Mulvenna, C., Hoad, C.L., Marciani, L., Barrett, D.A., Lomer, C.E., de Vos, W.M., Gowland, P.A. and Spiller, R.C. (2018, July 26). A low FODMAP diet is associated with changes in the microbiota and reduction in breath hydrogen but not colonic volume in healthy subjects. *PLoS One*, 13(7), e0201410. DOI: 10.1371/journal.pone.0201410.

Smith, R.N., Mann N.J., Braue, A., Mäkeläinen, H., and Varigos, G.A. (2007a, July). A low-glycemic-load diet improves symptoms in acne vulgaris patients: a randomized controlled trial. *Am J Clin Nutr*, 86(1), 107-115. DOI: 10.1093/ajcn/86.1.107

Smith, R.N., Mann, N.J., Braue, A., Mäkeläinen, H., and Varigos, G.A. (2007b, August). The effect of a high-protein, low glycemic-load diet versus a conventional, high glycemic-load diet on biochemical parameters associated with acne vulgaris: a randomized, investigator-masked, controlled trial. *J Am Acad Dermatol*, 57(2), 247-256. DOI: 10.1016/j.jaad.2007.01.046

Smith, R., Mann, N., Mäkeläinen, H., Roper, J., Braue, A., and Varigos, G. (2008, June). A pilot study to determine the short-term effects of a low glycemic load diet on hormonal markers of acne: a nonrandomized, parallel, controlled feeding trial. *Mol Nutr Food Res*, 52(6), 718-726. DOI: 10.1002/mnfr.200700307

Soliman, G.A. (2013, June 19). The role of mechanistic target of rapamycin (mTOR) complexes signaling in the immune responses. *Nutrients*, 5(6), 2231-2257. DOI: 10.3390/nu5062231.

Song, Y.C., Hahn, H.J., Kim, J.Y., Ko, J.H., Lee, Y.W., Choe, Y.B. and Ahn, K.J. (2011). Epidemiologic Study of *Malassezia* Yeasts in Acne Patients by Analysis of 26S rDNA PCR-RFLP. *Ann Dermatol*, 23, 321-328.

Sturniolo, G.C., Di Leo, V., Ferronato, A., D'Odorico, A. and D'Incà, R. (2001, May). Zinc supplementation tightens "leaky gut" in Crohn's disease. *Inflamm Bowel Dis*, 7(2), 94-98. DOI: 10.1097/00054725-200105000-00003.

Takagi, Y., Kaneda, K., Miyaki, M., Matsuo, K., Kawada, H. and Hosokawa, H. (2015). The long-term use of soap does not affect the pH-maintenance mechanism of human skin. *Skin Res Technol*, 21, 144-148. https://doi.org/10.1111/srt.12170

Takayasu, S., Wakimoto, H., Itami, S. and Sano, S. (1980, April). Activity of testosterone 5 alpha-reductase in various tissues of human skin. *J Invest Dermatol*, 74(4), 187-191. DOI: 10.1111/1523-1747.ep12541698.

Tanghetti, E.A. (2013, September). The role of inflammation in the pathology of acne. *J Clin Aesthet Dermatol*, 6(9), 27-35.

Treatment: Acne. (2017, September 21). NHS. https://www.nhs.uk/conditions/acne/treatment/

Tuohy, K., Brown, D., Klinder, A., Costabile, A. and Fava, F. (2010). Shaping the Human Microbiome with Prebiotic Foods – Current Perspectives for Continued Development. *Food Science and Technology Bulletin*, 7(4), 49-64. http://dx.doi.org/10.1616/1476-2137.15989

Vieth, R.F. and Sloan, H.R. (1986). A rotating unit for preparing circular chromatographic plates at elevated temperatures. *Journal of Chromatography A*, 357, 311-314.

Wang, B., Wu, G., Zhou, Z., Dai, Z., Sun, Y., Ji, Y., Li, W., Wang, W., Liu, C., Han, F. and Wu, Z. (2015, October). Glutamine and intestinal barrier function. *Amino Acids*, 47(10):2143-2154. DOI: 10.1007/s00726-014-1773-4.

Wang, C., Zhu, C., Shao, L., Ye, J., Shen, Y. and Ren, Y. (2019, June 24). Role of Bile Acids in Dysbiosis and Treatment of Nonalcoholic Fatty Liver Disease. *Mediators Inflamm*. DOI: 10.1155/2019/7659509.

Wang, J., Ghosh, S.S. and Ghosh, S. (2017, April 1). Curcumin improves intestinal barrier function: modulation of intracellular signaling, and organization of tight junctions. *Am J Physiol Cell Physiol*, 312(4), C438-C445. DOI: 10.1152/ajpcell.00235.2016.

Webster, G.F. (2005, August). The pathophysiology of acne. *Cutis*, 76(2 Suppl), 4-7. PMID: 16164150.

Webster, G.F. (1995). Inflammation in acne vulgaris. *J Am Acad Dermatol*, 33, 247-253.

Weiss, E. and Katta, R. (2017, October 31). Diet and rosacea: the role of dietary change in the management of rosacea. *Dermatol Pract Concept*, 7(4), 31-37. DOI: 10.5826/dpc.0704a08

What is HMD. (n.d.). HMD Heavy Metal Detox. https://www.detoxmetals.com

Wolcott, L. and Fahey, T. (2002, January 1). *The Metabolic Typing Diet: Customize Your Diet To: Free Yourself from Food Cravings: Achieve Your Ideal Weight; Enjoy High Energy and Robust Health; Prevent and Reverse Disease.* Chatsworth: Harmony Publishing.

Youn, S.H., Choi, C.W., Choi, J.W. and Youn, S.W. (2013). The skin surface pH and its different influence on the development of acne lesion according to gender and age. *Skin Res Technol*, 19, 131-136. https://doi.org/10.1111/srt.12023

Your guide to safer personal care products. (n.d.). EWG's Skin Deep. https://www.ewg.org/skindeep/

Zaenglein, A.L., Pathy, A.L., Schlosser, B.J., Alikhan, A., Baldwin, H.E., Berson, D.S., Bowe, W.P., Graber, E.M., Harper, J.C., Kang, S., Keri, J.E., Leyden, J.J., Reynolds, R.V., Silverberg, N.B., Steingold, L.F., Tollefson, M.M., Weiss, J.S., Dolan, N.C., Sagan, A.A., Stern, M., Boyer, K.M. and Bhushan, R. (2016, May). Guidelines of care for the management of acne vulgaris. *J Am Acad Dermatol*, 74(5), 945-973.e33. DOI: 10.1016/j.jaad.2015.12.037

Zarogoulidis, P., Lampaki, S., Turner, J.F., Huang, H., Kakolyris, S., Syrigos, K. and Zarogoulidis, K. (2014, December). mTOR pathway: A current, up-to-date mini-review (Review). *Oncol Lett*, 8(6), 2367-2370. DOI: 10.3892/ol.2014.2608.

ACKNOWLEDGEMENTS

I would like to thank Elise Abram for doing such an amazing job editing the book and making it even easier for the reader to follow.

I'd also like to thank Daniella Blechner for guiding the whole publication process and making it as smooth a process as possible.

Thank you to Paul Chek for taking time out from your busy schedule writing your own book series to write the Foreword to this book, and to all my teachers over the last 30 years, who have shown me the way.

Last, but definitely not least, thank you to all my clients over the years who have taken my advice on board and to those who have been a challenge to coach and have, therefore, helped me grow into a better practitioner.

Conscious Dreams
P U B L I S H I N G

Transforming diverse writers
into successful published authors

www.consciousdreamspublishing.com

authors@consciousdreamspublishing.com

Let's connect

www.ingramcontent.com/pod-product-compliance
Lightning Source LLC
Chambersburg PA
CBHW051714020426

42333CB00014B/989